A GOOD DEATH

A COUPLE'S JOURNEY

Laura Schmidt

Joe Pizzarello

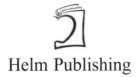

Helm Publishing

Copyediting: Dollie Parsons
Contributing editor: Norval G. Kennedy, MA, CT
Cover design: Robin Foster, Optima Design, Inc.
Layout: Pat Dodge, Pages Communications Service
Photos: Ralph Alswang, *Nightline*

Printed in the United States of America

Helm Publishing
213 Main Street/ P.O. Box 2105
Lake Dallas, TX 75065
940-497-3558 phone
940-497-2927 fax

Orders: 877-560-6025
www.helmpublishing.com
www.agooddeath.net

ISBN 0-9631033-9-3

Contents

Dedication

For Laura, my wife, partner and teacher:

Your compassion, dedication, and desire to help others
are an inspiration to us all. Through your words and
actions you have shown us how to find strength in adversity.
You live on through the valuable lessons you taught us.

Acknowledgments

We would like to thank the people who provided support and comfort
during difficult times, and those who assisted in making this book a reality.

John Pizzarello, Sr.

William Schmidt

Dr. Wayne Meyer

Julia McCrossin

John Driscoll

Robin Foster

Kathy Dietsch

Nancy Ochsenreiter

Dana Cable

Linda Dybiec

Bob and Pat Fry

Sara and Elliott Stoddard

Carolee Gearhart

Suzanne Rich

Joanne Lynn

Denise Watterson

Norval Kennedy

Dan Green

Kathy King

Introduction

Laura and I traveled the same path for more than 15 years. In early July 2003 we were secure in our marriage, had successful careers, and were surrounded by family and friends. Laura was approaching her 51st birthday, and I was coming up on my 50th. We had begun planning to travel to the coastal Carolinas and Georgia to explore relocation possibilities. We had decided that we were going to semi-retire in a few years. Laura was going to continue with her writing career, and I was going to look for part-time employment. We were going to play golf, travel and enjoy life together.

Our lives were changed forever when Laura was diagnosed with pancreatic cancer the day after her birthday and was given a prognosis of six to 12 months. In one heartbreaking instant, the path we were traveling became uncertain and scary. It would ultimately lead her to her death, and I would be left alone to continue on—not knowing where it would lead me.

Laura strongly believed in the importance of having what she called "a good death." Many factors led to her focusing her career on end-of-life issues. While taking care of her mother in the final months of her life, Laura had first-hand experience in dealing with doctors, Medicare, insurance companies and hospices. Working with hospice patients and their families, she saw the importance of effective communication between patients, their families and the medical professionals.

As a medical writer, Laura had worked in the end-of-life field for years, and at the time of her diagnosis she was in the process of completing her masters degree in thanatology—the study of death.

Even prior to her illness, Laura often said that too often treating the disease became more important than treating the patient and that the patients had little or no control over their treatment and, by extension, their lives. The reasons for this varied, but the common denominator was communication. Laura was a strong proponent of the use of health care power of attorney, living wills and advance directives, which provide a means for the patient to spell out his wishes for the end of his life.

As a society we are likely to prepare for the end of our lives by taking care of the business and financial issues. We usually prepare wills to safeguard and distribute our assets, and we buy life insurance to protect our families from financial hardship. Laura believed that identifying and communicating our wishes for our final days were of equal importance. Making one's desires known would give the families and caregivers of a dying patient a roadmap for dealing with the issues that might arise and provide the opportunity to make decisions consistent with the patient's wishes. This was the cornerstone for planning "a good death."

One of her core beliefs was that the time to deal with these issues is not when a crisis occurs, but at a point in time when they could be discussed honestly and rationally. Although we really don't like to envision our personal death, we need to make the decisions that will dictate the treatment that we will, or in some cases won't, receive at the end of our lives. The decision of whether we would want to be kept alive by respirators or feeding tubes is best made at a time when there is no pressure to make such a decision. It is for this reason that Laura and I had completed our living wills and advance directives and appointed each other as our health care power of attorney and reviewed everything periodically.

Laura decided to document her battle with cancer and write a book. This would be her final contribution to the end-of-life field. As a strong advocate for patients' rights, Laura wanted to get her message out. This book follows our journey down the path through both our perspectives—Laura's as a terminally ill cancer patient and mine as a caregiver and survivor.

1

I am Dying

I am dying. From the minute I received my diagnosis of pancreatic cancer three weeks ago, this has become my new identity. I am no longer the professional medical writer, the wife or the mother of our 93-pound golden retriever. All of a sudden, with the declaration of one sentence, I am someone new—someone whose physical health dominates over every other aspect of my life and defines my existence.

Receiving a diagnosis of terminal cancer has been the greatest shock of my life, but it isn't the diagnosis alone that has me paralyzed. It is the total change from being one way at one minute and then being something else the next. When a person receives a terminal diagnosis, it isn't just the end of his life. It is the end of that person's identity, character and feelings up to that point. The person who receives the diagnosis is not necessarily the same person who will go through the remaining days, and that is a frightening concept.

After the diagnosis, everything changes. I find that I doubt everything that I do and feel. After all, I thought I was healthy, so that is one major conception I had that was wrong. What else could be wrong? My actions, feelings and behaviors—they are all undergoing some sort of metamorphosis right now. Even though I have many family members and friends around for support, I realize that I am alone. Only I will die of this cancer. Only I will suffer. No words can describe how scared, isolated and anxious I am. My soul is shivering.

. . . .

2

Beginning the Journey

ex-pert 1. very skillful; having much training and knowledge in some special field. 2. of or from an expert (an expert opinion); 3. a person who is very skillful or highly trained and informed in some special field.—*Webster's Dictionary*

Some people deliberately choose a field of interest and become experts. Others, like myself, fall into this position quite by accident!

For 25 years I have worked as a freelance medical writer in the Washington, D.C. region, which is home to a wealth of prominent health care institutions in both the public and private sectors. Like an infant, my professional life was built by a series of small steps, each of which has put into place a firm foundation of knowledge and wisdom that only comes with time. Coupled with this is the influence of "the hand"—also known as the hand of God, the fickle finger of fate, destiny, or any other name. I believe that "the hand" guided me to my final destination: the study of death and dying.

When I was born, I had two grandparents, a mother and a father, and 20 aunts, uncles and cousins. Throughout the years, they all died—one by one at their appointed times—so by the time I celebrated my 50th birthday, the only ones left were my brothers and me.

Of all of the deaths that I experienced, certain ones stand out, like my grandmother's when I was 12 years old. She had a stroke two days before Christmas and lingered for three weeks in a coma-like state. I was amazed that death could be so peaceful and beautiful and that it could happen at any time, including Christmas! Years later, I held my aunt's hand as she slowly and methodically ... stopped ... breathing from lung cancer. *How mechanical death is*, I thought. And then there was my mother's death, so difficult and painful in many ways, which had a huge impact not only on me personally, but professionally as well.

. . . .

From the time I was born, all I knew was that I was a writer. But a writer of what? Although I was a published poet before I graduated from Marymount Manhattan College in New York City in 1976 with a Bachelor of Arts in English, I still had no idea what I was going to do with my life. Few people made any kind of money writing poetry. So I decided to pursue a master's program in journalism at American University in Washington, D.C., in the hopes that I would find my way professionally. But as soon as I signed a lease on an apartment, I learned that the school had overbooked the class, and I was deferred for six months.

Because I was financially tied to the area, I decided to go to a temporary agency for work, and my first assignment was as a secretary in the Pediatrics Department at Georgetown University Medical Center. This was the first time I was exposed to the "other side" of the health care arena—one where I wasn't a patient—and I found it fascinating and appealing. The only bad part, I thought, was that there was no place for my writing skills, so I didn't consider medicine as a career.

This feeling changed when a writing job in the hospital's public relations department opened up, and I applied for it. This was the unofficial beginning of my writing career in the medical arena, and I threw myself into learning everything I could about the mechanics of health care. Learning about writing in the health care field taught me how to market medical services, produce general-interest articles, and research peer-reviewed technical pieces—all the basics of health care communications.

Throughout all of this "training," I came into contact with patients, their family members and medical staff. Because I am an emotional person, it became important for me to learn how to distance myself from each case. I believed that I couldn't get too involved with the human aspects of medicine if I were to do my job as a writer correctly. So, like doctors and nurses, I learned to put up a defensive wall around myself and took the clinical point of view in dealing with sick people.

Specialization became the buzzword in the 1980s, and just as doctors and nurses were beginning to focus on specific areas of medicine, so too were medical writers. As the editor of *The Counselor* magazine for the National Association of Alcoholism and Drug Abuse Counselors in Arlington, Virginia, I learned not only about new approaches to treatment of alcoholics and drug addicts, but, more importantly, I became exposed to the pharmaceutical aspects of care. Understandably, morphine, fentanyl, oxycontin and other drugs of choice of addicts were negative influences in this arena, but in a different setting (such as a cancer patient's home), I could see how valuable they could be. This exposure to pain medications and their potential benefits was laying the foundation for my future writing on death and dying.

This interest in pain medications segued very nicely with my writing when I began my training as a cancer information specialist for the National Cancer Institute. In addition to intensely studying symptoms, prognoses and treatments for all major cancers, I had to apply this knowledge in the cancer field, corresponding with patients, family members and doctors. To fully understand what the cancer patients were going through, in 1997, I decided to become involved with hospice as a volunteer where I worked with diverse patients, many of whom had cancer, and their family members.

But a major turning point for me occurred when my own mother became seriously ill in 1998 with congestive heart failure. During the last six months of her life, I put my career on hold and played the role of primary caregiver, putting me on "the other side of the fence." This experience was invaluable as I got to see modern end-of-life care from the patient's perspective, and I was very disappointed. Poor communications, lack of coordination between hospice and her doctors, and the inability to meet—or even identify—her dying needs all fueled my anger and disgust at the current health care system.

I helped my mother die. No, not in the Kevorkian way of administering drugs to alleviate a painful end. Instead, my husband and I brought her into our house after her surgery. We chose to take care of her and provide her with comfort and companionship until it was her time to go.

We were prepared to deal with the constant turmoil associated with a terminal illness—the uncertainty and anxiety, financial burdens, the midnight runs to the pharmacy, the sometimes incompetent home care aides, even the loss of personal privacy. Our lives were built around doctors' visits and prescription refills as her illness dominated our household. What made it all worthwhile was that at the end, we had accomplished our goal. My mother died in a comfortable room, surrounded by people who truly loved her, with no cold floors, intravenous lines or frightening medical equipment around.

• • • • • • • • • • • • • • • • • • •

Surprisingly, quite a few people we talked to, including Mom's doctor, felt she should go straight to a nursing home to reduce the burden on us and the physician. Joe and I could not begin to comprehend the thought. When did nursing homes become replacements for love and family loyalty?

At my insistence, my mother was finally admitted to hospice care five days before she died. The doctor's justification for allowing hospice was that it would be easier to deal with her medical condition. Hospice care is built on the concept that the patient can die in the comfort of his or her home, and this was our intention, and Mom's wish. Hospice is not available to make the doctor's job easier. This is one of the falsehoods that some in the medical profession carry about hospice care.

I do believe that nursing homes have a valuable place in our society and in our lives. They can provide care and rehabilitation for those who are alone, or who need specialized care. However, in the case of a terminally ill person, they should not be accepted as "the easy way out" of a painful family situation. Many families in today's society are constantly moving farther away from each other in an attempt to move up the corporate ladder. The down side to this tunnel vision on career is that many times the adult children are not in a position to help a terminally ill parent. Unfortunately, for many of these patients, nursing homes have become "families by default."

Although it is perfectly acceptable for a new mother or father to take time off from work to concentrate on the first months of their infant's life, many people are uncomfortable with helping a dying parent end his or her life comfortably within the confines of a loving home. Even though most people say they wish for this kind of end to their lives, the sad reality is that many die in places other than their homes. It is a sad reflection that nursing homes are perceived as the perfect replacement for love, companionship and intimacy that only a family can have.

Just as all of us are concerned with and see the value of ensuring that a child has a good solid beginning in life, filled with love and guidance, so too should we try to help people nearing the end of their life cycle. Death is a natural part of life. There is nothing wrong with bringing it into one's own home.

After my mother died in November 1998, I decided to become more involved in this specialized health care field, and I wanted to learn everything I could about death and the dying process. Rather than turn my back disgust-

· · · · · · · · · · · · · · · · · · · ·

edly on the end-of-life field, I chose to funnel my anger towards the *hospice* and *palliative care* fields in positive ways. (Hospices offer care at many levels for the dying patient and families. You will find more information about hospice in later chapters. Palliative care specifically tries to keep the dying patient comfortable, notably controlling excessive pain.) With this focus, I learned:

- the business side of hospice from the National Hospice and Palliative Care Organization;
- the political side of palliative care from Last Acts, a national coalition of 1,000 health care institutions;
- and the human side of palliative care from the grassroots organization, Americans for Better Care of the Dying.

To augment this work, I decided in 2001 to get my Master of Arts in Thanatology degree from Hood College in Frederick, Maryland. I thought this academic focus on the studies of death and dying would enhance my writing and give me a firm foundation for writing about the issues and challenges that lay before the field.

With all of this background—as a professional medical writer, hospice volunteer, primary caregiver, and student—I had the experience, education and credentials to call myself an expert in end-of-life care. Little did I know that all of these efforts were only practice for my future work—as a dying patient.

"Are you telling me I'm dying?"
With tears in his eyes, my doctor nodded his head in a silent "yes."

Now it is my turn. And the irony of my situation and its link to my personal and professional background is uncanny. From the minute I learned there was a cancer growing in my body, my role as a dying person became my new identity. All of a sudden, with the declaration of one sentence, I am someone new—someone whose physical demise dominates over every other aspect of my life and defines my existence. And all the while, the clock is ticking towards an unknown, but near, time when I will cease to exist.

. . . .

For many people like myself, death and dying become all too real within a single poignant moment. In that short exchange with my doctor, I went from the land of the living to the land of the dying, a place most healthy people in society choose not to think about.

Up to the moment of my diagnosis, I was a seemingly healthy midlife woman. My yearly physical showed that I was in good shape for a 50-year-old, and husband Joe and I had begun talking enthusiastically about putting an addition on our house, a cruise the next year, and retirement plans. In short, we were looking forward to the future and growing old together.

But everything changed on a Friday afternoon in June 2003. I was in the middle of finishing my coursework for my master's degree when I decided that the stress was too great. Sitting in a classroom every weekend was beginning to hurt my lower back, so I made an appointment to have a nice, relaxing massage.

During the course of the massage, I remember thinking how rough the massage therapist was, and I was very happy (for once) to have the session end; however, I wasn't prepared for the surprise I found the next morning when I saw that my lower back was black and blue. More importantly, I was in tremendous pain that radiated down both sides of my back.

I didn't let that stop me, however, and I went to class the next day, armed with the ice bricks that are used in packing lunches. Periodically, I would put an ice brick on one side of my back, and when that side was numb, move the brick to the other side. But the pain defied the ice packs, and for the first time in my life, I walked out of class.

Joe and I discussed going to the emergency room, but we dismissed this idea because we thought he would get charged with domestic abuse. What else could cause such terrible bruising? So I waited until Monday to see my regular doctor, Dr. Wayne Meyer whose office is in Rockville, Maryland. Having been a patient of his for a number of years, Dr. Meyer was used to me coming in for unusual problems, such as my pernicious anemia. So this episode just fell into that class of "unusual" as Dr. Meyer documented the bruises and put me on muscle relaxers and pain medication.

"You'll be fine in a week," he said casually.

* * * * * * * * * * * * * * * * * * *

One week later, the bruises had faded but the pain remained undiminished. For the next three Mondays, I went to Dr. Meyer, anxious to find the cause of the pain. Although an MRI found no sign of a ruptured disc, there was evidence of a damaged sciatic nerve. But would that be enough to cause such intense pain?

Finally, Dr. Meyer decided to be more aggressive and put me on steroids to help calm the inflammation. But as soon as I woke up the next morning, I was paralyzed with pain. In addition to the radiating pain in my back, now there were new sharp pains in my stomach. The best description I can give (which women can relate to) is that it felt like having the worst gas on the first day of your worst menstrual period!

That Monday—ironically my 51st birthday—Dr. Meyer ordered a CAT scan to check on my gallbladder as a possible source for the pain. The CAT scan was scheduled for 7:30 a.m. the next day, and by 9:15 a.m. Tuesday, Dr. Meyer's office called, asking that I come to the office that afternoon.

"Be sure to bring your husband with you," nurse Debbie said.

I knew something was up. My health care training taught me that there was a sense of urgency from this phone call. And to insist that Joe come too told me that the doctor felt I needed support to hear bad news. *This is ridiculous*, I thought to myself. *It's only my gallbladder. Nothing life-threatening. Just an annoying surgery.* That is all Joe and I were focusing on—my gallbladder. It never occurred to us that anything else could be wrong!

But when we arrived at the doctor's office for the appointment, our combined antennae were up. Neither the receptionist nor the nurse would even look at us, and there were no other patients in the waiting area.

"Remember that scene in 'The Godfather' when Sonny goes up to the toll booth?" Joe whispered to me, alluding to the massacre that killed the godfather's hotheaded son. "I feel as if we're at the toll booth right now." While we both laughed, we didn't realize the prophetic nature of Joe's comments.

As soon as we entered the examination room, Dr. Meyer came in, CAT scan films in hand.

* * * * * * * * * * * * * * * * * *

"Your gallbladder is fine," he said, "but there is plenty of bad news. You have a tumor in the tail of your pancreas, and the cancer has already spread to your liver and lung." I looked at him dumbfounded, as if he were talking about someone else. I went into that emotional twilight zone where nothing is real or concrete.

He went on to explain that the CAT scan showed the tumor accounted for about one third of the pancreas, and there were multiple lesions on my liver and lung. Shaped like a fish with a wide head, a tapering body, and a narrow pointed tail, the pancreas is six inches long and less than two inches wide. Diagnosing pancreatic cancer is difficult because the organ is located behind the stomach, making the pancreas invisible to traditional x-rays. My tumor in the tail of this "fish" meant that the tumor was on the left side of the pancreas next to my spleen, and the first place the cancer usually spreads is to the liver.

"There was no way of knowing that the tumor was there unless it was found by accident like this," said Dr. Meyer. The whole time he was talking, I was craning my neck to make sure that it really was *my name* on the CAT scan film.

What makes pancreatic cancer so bad is that it is a silent killer. Like most of the other 30,700 pancreatic cancer patients diagnosed in 2003, I hadn't experienced any symptoms, despite the advanced state of the cancer.[1] Looking back, the only tip-off was that I had been losing weight—16 pounds during the previous six months—but I, like many other women of my age, attributed any bodily changes to menopause. Most symptoms of pancreatic cancer, such as pain and nausea, become apparent only when it is too late to go for a potential cure. In my case, it was too late.

I sat in silent shock as Joe began asking a million questions. With my background as a trained cancer-information specialist, I didn't have to ask any questions. I knew what Dr. Meyer was telling me—that I had between six and 12 months to live. But despite my knowledge of the disease and its prognosis for the future, I still had to have my worst fear confirmed. That is when Dr. Meyer and I had our poignant "eye-to-eye" moment.

As the truth began to hit me, I slumped over, repeating, "Oh my God," over and over again. For the first minute or so, I was so numb by the news that I couldn't process or react to anything. I couldn't even cry! Joe, however, be-

• • • • • • • • • • • • • • • • • • • •

came so upset that he fell off the examination table he was sitting on. It wasn't until we hugged that I let go of my emotions, and together, we began to cry hysterically. Even Dr. Meyer was still crying. After a couple of minutes, I abruptly announced that I had to leave the doctor's office.

"It's nothing personal, Dr. Meyer," I said. "I just have to get out of here."

I was too overwhelmed, shocked and crying. It was simply too painful for me to deal with. Never in my wildest dreams would I have thought that I had cancer. Pushing any ideas of death aside, I was emotionally dealing just with the cancer aspect, and my mind was racing through what lay ahead: treatment, physical changes, and possible surgery. My fears of dealing with my gallbladder were nothing compared to what I was feeling now. I just wanted to run far away and pretend that these past few minutes hadn't occurred. Each minute was becoming too unbearable, and I went into complete emotional shutdown.

With his usual compassion, Dr. Meyer didn't try to stop me or want to talk—he simply opened the door ... and we ran. Because the elevator in the building tends to be slow, Joe and I went into the stairwell and, between floors, hugged each other for what seemed like hours.

"Our lives are over," Joe said quietly.

No amount of education, training, work experience or personal loss can prepare a person for his or her own death. When the diagnosis is given, the dying process becomes "new ground," and each person responds in individual and unique ways.

Quite frankly, in dealing with my own pending demise, the stakes of understanding death and dying have become much higher. Nowhere is this better demonstrated than when I was first approached to be on ABC TV's *Nightline*. The format for the show called for me to be interviewed twice: once as an "expert" in the end-of-life field and then, later, as a dying person. Film crews followed Joe and me everywhere for three weeks: to my doctor's office, to chemo, to an MRI and to our home.

What became quickly apparent to me during this time was there was no definitive line of when I was the "expert" and when I was the dying person. Rather, *I was the expert because I was dying.* My professional and academic background played little role in positioning me as the "expert." My credentials

. . . .

were not based on academic or professional achievement. Rather, they were based on the fact that only a dying person such as myself can know the intricacies, challenges and fears that accompany the dying process. While my work taught me the right words to say, my role as the terminally ill patient reflected the feelings, observations and perspectives about the dying process. Until you are in the position of being the dying person, there is no way you can truly know what the dying process is like. And because the dying process is so individualistic, each dying person is the expert on his or her own death.

Dying Patients in Modern Health Care

But few people—in the health care field, in society or even dying patients—realize the patient is the expert. While attention has focused on caregivers and others involved in the end-of-life field, the dying patient—the one who is lying in the bed and is scared and lonely—has fallen through the cracks of modern health care. Dying patients in the early part of the twenty-first century do not receive the same care, respect and attention that other participants in the end-of-life maze receive. Instead, considerable focus is being placed on educating physicians and other medical professionals on end-of-life issues, working with insurance companies to increase benefits and providing caregivers with training, knowledge and support. This attention is the result of the need *for all people* on end-of-life concerns.

But what about the dying person? What is being done to help the terminally ill reach peace and contentment at the end of life? Perhaps people think that medical professionals, insurance executives, caregivers and dying people are one in the same in that they share a common goal of trying to provide at the end of life. But in reality, they are not. Giving support to one group does not necessarily benefit the other.

I have seen a few "good deaths." *But more often, I have been appalled by the many "bad deaths" in our society—those where key issues such as inadequate pain management, ignored patient wishes, loneliness and isolation have dictated a dying patient's final days and minutes.* Having a "good" death should be easy to achieve in our sophisticated and expansive society, but it is not. As a result, many terminally ill patients are suffering needlessly.

. . . .

So this book will hopefully give a voice to the terminally ill patient. This book is based on my experiences, and I hope that readers will gain insight into what dying people go through during their final days so that support and care can match their desperate and profound needs. In addition, it is the intention of this book to empower the terminally ill in their roles as experts in the end-of-life arena.

Lessons Learned: Diagnosis

- The dying person is the true expert on death and dying. This role empowers patients to be active participants in care and treatment planning as well as defining unique needs that must be met in order to have "a good death."
- When the diagnosis of terminal illness is first given, the patient's initial reaction is usually anxiety, not depression.
- It is appropriate and normal for everyone involved in the initial meeting—physicians, patients and family members—to show emotion upon hearing the diagnosis. By sharing feelings at this vulnerable time, a special and exceptionally strong bond can be created between the medical professional and the patient that lays the foundation for a trusting relationship.
- Because the diagnosis is overwhelming, don't overload the patient with too much information at the beginning. Give the person time and space to absorb this huge shock.
- Let the patient dictate the initial discussion of the illness. Don't try and force conversation if the patient isn't psychologically prepared to accept it. If the patient wants to leave without knowing everything, that is okay.
- The initial consultation does not have to deal with everything related to the illness and treatment. A second follow-up meeting a couple of days later might give the patient and any family members the right amount of time to start adjusting to the illness and more capably consider options.

. . . .

- Be aware that from the moment of diagnosis, the person will undergo a change of self-identity. In order to "survive" both physically and socially, the person must adapt to a society that shuns death. The person that you talk to at the beginning of the illness might not be the same person towards the end.
- Call the person the next day just to see how he/she is doing No one should go through the initial phase of a terminal illness alone! A two-second phone call by the physician lets the person know that someone is on his side and available for support: "Hello. I am thinking about you."
- Dying people have unique needs that must be addressed. Yet too often these needs are ignored and misunderstood as concentration in the end-of-life field is focusing on the other partners in the dying process: medical professionals, insurance companies and caregivers. *Do not assume that what is being done for those groups in terms of education and support will automatically filter down to the dying patient.*

• • • • • • • • • • • • • • • • • •

3

Responding to the News

The presence of death evokes all kinds of emotions and reactions simply because it is one of nature's universal common elements. Just as each of us is born, so too, must we die.

But just because death is a natural part of life doesn't make it any easier to accept or understand. Whether dealing with it in spiritual, scientific or even practical terms, death is frightening because it is mysterious and threatening. Not only does it highlight potential loss and pain, but death also reminds us of our personal mortality. It is one of the few elements in life that unites all of us in one collective community, allowing us to share in each death.

These feelings of apprehension don't apply just to ourselves, our family and close friends when they die. Because we are all part of the same living community, losing someone who is not personally known to us can be equally traumatic. For example, I can remember when John Lennon died. Being a true baby boomer, I felt as if I grew up with John through his music, and I spent many teenage years being entertained and comforted by him. While I never met him, my sense of loss—a feeling that is shared by many fans—brought death closer to me. "If he could die, then I can too," I thought to myself. Although my feelings over losing him are not as intense and personal as when my mother died, his passing did bring out the fear, confusion and terror that go along with today's perception of death and dying.

So, when a diagnosis of terminal illness is given, the impact from the news doesn't affect just the patient. It affects everyone's mortality. But how this translates out into general society is challenging, to say the least. Today's society prides itself on being open and free, and people are willing to talk about everything: sex, violence, and personal finances. But the one thing they won't talk about is death. This presents a dilemma to all of us in the collective community because how can you deal with something if you won't even talk about it?

• •

Instead of dying at home surrounded by loved ones, terminally ill patients in 2003 are placed in hospitals and nursing homes because that is where proper care using sophisticated equipment can be given. This makes it easy to "put the person away" so the family doesn't have to deal with the harsh emotions related to death and loss. It also creates the illusion that the person might not die because of the close proximity to medical care.

The impact of this massive change in acceptance has forced many terminally ill patients onto the "back burner" of medical care where their needs are not met and their existence is frequently not even acknowledged. Bob was a hospice patient who died of emphysema alone in a dark-lit hospital room. The medical staff came in only to give him pain medications, and, despite having a wife, daughter and three grandchildren, there was no one to comfort him in his final minutes.

Medical technical advances have also taken the focus of the death from being a spiritual life event and molded it into a cost-driven financial consideration. Whereas in previous years, families would pay for their loved one's illness and death, these expensive costs—and the rising cost of health care in general—are now subject to oversight by managed care, insurance companies and Medicare. By doing so, the patient loses control over her life and death in an effort by insurance companies and hospitals to dictate coverage merely to save money.

In addition, the funeral industry has benefited from this denial of death. People who are denying death don't want either themselves or their loved ones to look like they are dead. *Millions of dollars are spent each year on elaborate funerals and burial rituals whose pomp and glamour frequently mask the true reality of the death.*

As a result of these massive changes, death is no longer seen as a "beautiful ritual." Rather, it is a technical and frequently ugly event, leaving the dying person to be alone, isolated and forgotten.

Medical professionals too have changed their perceptions of death. Rather than seeing it as a natural part of the life cycle, as in previous centuries, doctors and nurses now see death as a failure—of the medical field, of technology and of their own personal skills. It challenges their godlike status. *What doctors don't realize is that when a patient dies, it is not their failure. Rather, it is the individual's body that has failed!*

• • • • • • • • • • • • • • • • • • •

The current end-of-life atmosphere is in a Catch-22 cycle. Rather than concentrate on the terminally ill patient's desperate needs, attention is focused on prognostication (how long someone will live) and its impact on policy and personal/professional concerns. To access Medicare or any other insurance benefit covering terminal illness, the responsibility lies on the physician to give an accurate prognosis. Too often, the difficulty and uncertainty in doing so might carry a punitive element that backlashes on the doctor (and the medical field as a whole).

This underlying threat impedes not only the health care perception of death, making it more financially oriented rather than care centered, but, via the trickle-down effect, society's view of death as natural is skewed to deny death at any expense.

The Patient's Reactions

So what does this reflection on society's view of the dying process have to do with my death? Plenty! These perspectives have the potential to influence every aspect of my life from the kind of care I am receiving to how I am accepted by my friends. But regardless of this harsh picture, I have found that new changes in attitude are slowly occurring. Despite the denial of death that is rampant on the national level, death and dying are more accepted and acknowledged on the individual levels. Sometimes it just takes a while to come to the surface.

My reaction to my diagnosis is a prime example of what I mean. For the first two weeks after learning that I was dying, I was in shock. Whenever anyone started talking about cancer, I would excuse myself and go to bed. In retrospect, I think it is interesting that I reverted to my childhood during this time. As an adult, I always sleep on my back or my side—never my stomach. But after the diagnosis, I would automatically lie on my stomach and cover my head with my arms. Each time, it reminded me of a newborn baby lying in a crib. I guess it was my version of assuming the fetal position when threatened!

During those times when I couldn't "take to my bed" like Scarlett O'Hara, I would simply tune out any conversation regarding my health. As a medical writer, I usually wanted to know every detail and procedure related to an illness. But with me as the patient, I found I didn't want to know a thing regarding my health—and this included the extent of the cancer spread.

· · · · · · · · · · · · · · · · · ·

"Don't tell me anymore," I told Dr. Kenneth Miller, my oncologist, cutting him short in his report on my cancer. "I'm on overload."

The truth is, learning where my cancer had spread was too painful to hear. This inability on my part to deal with reality put an even heavier importance on Joe to be my eyes and ears when talking to the doctors. But what we found was Joe was just as overwhelmed; he, too, frequently missed valuable information and was confused about what was to come. So we began to bring a tape recorder with us as a backup so that no bit of information would be lost between the doctors and us. Looking back, it would have been helpful if a third person, such as a good friend, were with us.

Even though the health care field emphasizes bringing your significant other or a family member along to a medical appointment, I think many people would react as Joe did. If the person is too emotionally involved with the patient, the rules that apply to the patient's inability to comprehend automatically spill over onto the loved one. Having a third party who is not that involved would ensure that the crucial information is relayed to the patient and family at the best time (probably out of the doctor's office).

During the first two weeks, I found myself questioning every belief and principle that had governed my life so far. Because life had just dealt me a tremendously difficult blow, I no longer could trust anyone or anything. Is there a God? Do Heaven and Hell really exist? What happens after death? Despite my firm spiritual beliefs and extensive education in the death-and-dying field, I felt as if everything were "new" and uncertain. This doubt created a special kind of suffering for me as I felt, for the first time in my life, scared of everything and everyone, including God.

But I think this was just part of the shock phase in the dying process. When I was able to accept the fact that I had cancer (not that I was dying), I gradually returned to my old beliefs and principles. That is not to say that I was not scared of dying—I was—but at least, I could put it into a context that I could deal with better.

Dealing with cancer and dealing with death are two distinct concepts for a dying person. Cancer, or any other terminal illness, brings its own fears and worries that are separate from its final result. "I can't believe I have cancer," is a line I repeated over and over again, without giving any thought to death.

•   •   •   •   •   •   •   •   •   •   •   •   •   •   •   •   •   •

Instead, I was thinking of chemotherapy, radiation, pain, possible surgery, and all of the medical characteristics that are part of the disease. I was trying to understand the impact the cancer was going to have on my life, such as quitting working, without any concern about how cancer would influence my death.

Once a certain level of acceptance and understanding was achieved regarding the disease, I was able to move on to conceptualizing death. "I can't believe I'm dying. I can't believe I'm going through this." In dealing with death issues, it made no difference to me if death were due to cancer or any other disease. The simple fact that I was dying emotionally paralyzed me. One of the first major tasks of any dying patient is to integrate "cause and result" as a way to have a full picture of the situation. But this might not happen for a long time because each component—the disease and the death—is so overwhelming and frightening on its own.

Some of my friends asked, "What is it like to know you are dying?" And my answer so far has been, "When I know, I'll tell you." But the truth of the matter is that the knowledge impacts on every action and every thought in every day. In a certain respect, knowing that I am dying is just as bad as having the cancer. It is pervasive, insulting and absolutely terrifying.

When I start to panic, I try to make myself think about all those people who die suddenly and who don't have the time to say good-bye or finish their life's work. While I'm not volunteering to go through this phase of my life, I am grateful that I do have the opportunity to do something with my last days.

Whenever I become depressed or despondent over my current situation, I try to mentally and emotionally reframe it. For me, dying suddenly and without warning would not give me the control over my life that I would like at the end. While pain and suffering are not what anyone would choose at the time of death, my personal option would be to have the opportunity to say good-bye to my loved ones and to finish the life projects that I feel are important.

These days, I often think of Alice D., who was the nurse at the hospital when my mother was first diagnosed with congestive heart failure. My mother's 77-year-old body started to show circulatory problems, and she decided to have major surgery so that she could walk again. But in the operating room, her heart and her lungs gave out because of the stress of the procedure. By the time Mom made it into the recovery room, her doctors told us that she was dying.

. . . .

During Mom's month-long stay in the hospital, Alice was her primary nurse, a peppy and very attractive redhead who truly loved her job. At age 38, she was the mother of five children, had a strong marriage and was a very devout Christian. When Mom was discharged from the hospital, Alice went over her medication regimen with me and helped me get over the panic of being a primary caregiver. When Mom and I left the hospital, all of the knowledge that I had came from Alice, and she said that I could call her anytime with questions. Nevertheless, I was terrified of my new role as caregiver.

Not long after Mom was discharged from the hospital, an alleged drunken driver's car hit the car carrying Alice, her husband and their kids, which instantly killed both parents and three of the children. Her story was on the front page of the newspaper because of the horror of the accident. That is where I learned that Alice came to nursing late in life. In fact, she had been a nurse for only a few years. Prior to that, she had been lost and without purpose in her life. But she pulled herself together, met the man of her dreams, had the kids, and found a career in nursing. What an accomplishment for her! And it was when she had done all of the things necessary to complete her life's lesson that she died.

I don't think any of us know what our life's lessons are, but I do believe that we are each given the opportunity to realize our full potential. Especially when facing the final days of my life, the realization that there is a higher power or God who is in ultimate control over my life makes me appreciate life as being a partnership between each of us and God. This attitude has given me the strength to face each day now, and it is a major part of my coping mechanisms, especially during a difficult time like this.

The Caregiver's Reaction

In contrast to my "leave me alone" attitude, Joe's reaction to my illness began with anger. He was furious with Dr. Meyer, life and God for "giving Laura a death sentence." When we left Dr. Meyer's office immediately after the diagnosis, Joe began yelling in the parking lot about how it was so unfair, and "Why did this happen?" He became so overwrought that he doesn't even remember driving home that day.

* * * * * * * * * * * * * * * * * * * *

Once the shock wore off, Joe became like a robot, dealing with issues on a practical and masculine basis. "I call myself the 'Make a Wish Foundation,'" he said. "Whatever Laura or the doctors want, I make it happen." This appearance of being on autopilot, which I think is a very masculine trait, also translated over to his emotional side. Because we had his father staying with us, it was difficult for both Joe and me to freely express our emotions and fears. In Joe's case, he frequently expressed his emotions through anger and temper tantrums over the slightest things, and the anger was usually directed at his father. Even after his father went back home, Joe's primary emotion was anger. Even now, only in our darkest moments will he allow himself to cry and show fear. Trying to emotionally protect me, he tries very hard not to show me his panic and depression, so he often takes a long shower where he closes the door and cries.

Joe's Thoughts

When Laura asked Dr. Meyer if she were dying, my mind went numb. It was total mental paralysis. A million thoughts were swirling around in my head, but I was unable to land on a cohesive thought. I was glad when Laura said we were leaving because the room was getting claustrophobic.

When we arrived home I remember talking to Laura about what the next steps were going to be. Dr. Meyer's office was going to get her a referral to see an oncologist, and I kept telling Laura that we shouldn't jump to any rash conclusions. After all, at that point what we didn't know was more than we did know. I was trying to keep up a strong front, but it wasn't a convincing act. The thought that Laura might die within the next year was something I couldn't deal with. I couldn't imagine my life without her. I wasn't in denial—I was terrified!

The only thing I knew for certain was that whatever the future held, Laura and I were going to go through it together. She was beginning the toughest time of her life, and I was going to be there with her to do whatever I could to support her.

Other People's Reactions

Both Joe and I are very open people. Being Italian, I think it's part of our character makeup to talk about everything, and this sharing of thoughts and feelings has evolved into one of our marriage's strongest coping mechanisms. When we learned of my diagnosis, our approach to dealing with it (at least on the surface) was no different.

After a long discussion about who should and should not be told, both of us realized that it was foolish to withhold the truth from anyone. Not only was my body going to change considerably over the next months, but our behaviors and daily routines would make the cancer presence even more apparent to others.

In addition, my reasons for telling people came from a different and deeper level. Having worked in the end-of-life field for 12 years and nearing the end of my studies for a master's in thanatology, I knew first hand about society's denial of death. People don't like to think about death, let alone talk about it, and now being in the position of a terminally ill patient, I could see how this silence and avoidance hurts those who are suffering so much already. How unfair and unkind to abandon someone at this crucial and painful time!

Because Joe and I were honest with people regarding my condition, I was forcing an atmosphere of open awareness, whether the other people liked it or not. What they did and how they reacted after the initial acknowledgement was up to them, but at least we presented a situation that was sincere, truthful and human, albeit very painful.

Although we were apprehensive about how people would react, we began to tell people about my cancer: not just close friends and relatives, but everyone with whom we came in regular contact. Our feeling was that if the person couldn't deal with it, it was his or her problem, not ours. We had enough of our own. But to our surprise, this was rarely the case. In fact, the reactions to my illness were truly overwhelming and inspiring.

For example, I went to my vet's to pick up pills for our dog. Because the animal hospital was very busy, I just put the check down on the counter and walked out with the medication. Halfway into the parking lot, I hear my name being called. Thinking I made the check out wrong, I turn around and there was Sue, who at age 22 is the youngest person working at the hospital. Sue

· · · · · · · · · · · · · · · · · · · ·

comes over to me, gives me a big hug and starts crying on my shoulder. We stood there for about two minutes until she turned to go back to work. Not one word was said during this entire time, but I felt her compassion, support and love.

At the grocery store, I ran into my favorite cashier, Geri, and during the course of our conversation, I mentioned my cancer. She, too, gave me a big hug and then proceeded to tell me about her 29-year-old brother's death from bone cancer the year before. In fact, the conversation turned so emotional that she decided to take a break, and we sat on a bench outside the store for half an hour talking about death, dying and grief. At the end of our talk, she said that was the first time since his death that she had talked about him. Not only did both of us feel better at the end of our talk, but a special bond was created between us that afterward was evident every time I walked into the store.

Sometimes talking about death can produce some surprising information as I found out when some relatives came to visit. Because I didn't know them very well, the conversation started out being very "polite," talking about the weather and other casual topics. The tone of the conversation changed when one cousin, Larry, turned to me and said, "I don't know if this is out of line or not, but is chemo really as bad as they say?" That question gave the opening to everyone to talk not only about my cancer, and what Joe and I were going through, but it unwittingly gave each cousin the opportunity to think about and map out a living will, beginning with, "If I were in your shoes ..." When everyone got up to leave, Larry pulled me aside. "I face death everyday, just like you," he said. "I have such a bad heart that the doctor says that each day is a gift. But I don't talk to my family about my fears and anxiety. This discussion really helped me." For the first time in a long while, I realized that I wasn't the only dying person. Leave it to the "other one" to start this valuable discussion on death.

For me personally, the greatest reaction I received was from my father-in-law, John Pizzarello. A widower who lives in Florida, Dad packed his bags and came to our house to help take care of me. For the first three months, Dad made my breakfast and lunch, and he kept me company during the day. The reason why this was so special to me was because my own father died more than 30 years ago. I was never close to my father, and in my father-in-law, I

. . . .

found the father I always wanted. The sacrifice this 77-year-old man made for me is the perfect example of words and actions coming together. It helped this dying person to know that people loved me and were willing to help me during this difficult time.

Even those whom we expect to be compassionate and accepting of death can also show a deeper understanding of what it takes to die. When Joe and I attended the annual awards dinner at the Hospice Network of Maryland in November 2003, I knew I was going to be surrounded by hospice and palliative care professionals, those people who see death every day.

Hospice Caring had nominated me for the, "You Make A Difference" award, and as a recipient, I had to go up to the dais when my name was called (Joe had to help me because I was so weak), and stand next to the executive director who read my biography to the audience. Doing this was very difficult for me because the biography laid my life out in black and white, and the mention of my cancer became a "reality" moment. I didn't want to show any emotion, however, because I thought I was in the midst of all of these professionals who were calm and collected. Was I wrong! I received a standing ovation from the 250 participants and many people in the room began crying. The auras of love, empathy and reaching out were overwhelming, and I ran to the bathroom to have a good cry. Walking back to my table, every "professional" became a personal friend, sharing good wishes and prayers with me. The evening was one of the highlights of my life, one that shows even the people who deal with death daily never get used to its presence.

What I have learned from my experiences is that people *want* to talk about and deal with death. Healthy people want to know more as a way of dealing with personal loss. I think it is part of the "sharing in the social community" that psychoanalysis and other theories of therapy talk about. Dying people, too, want to talk about death. By being open and honest, a dying person gains strength, support and love from many sources, often unexpectedly.

* * * * * * * * * * * * * * * * * * *

Negative Reactions

Of course, many reactions to my health were painful, insensitive and uncomfortable. A friend of mine told me that her brother-in-law had just been diagnosed with prostate cancer.

"The doctors say they can get it all, and he won't even need chemo," she said. "Thank God, he isn't as bad off as you are. Your cancer is so much worse."

I was quite surprised when negative reactions came from other cancer patients. I was sitting in the chemo room, having blood work done, when the man across the room began talking to me.

"My chemo is a breeze," he said. "I have no side effects and just have to take this one bag once a week."

"You're lucky," I responded. "I have five bags of chemo that I get every two weeks and the side effects are just awful. The nausea is particularly bad."

"Well, you know what they say—we get what we deserve. I guess my karma is better than yours ... and my chemo is working!"

How do you respond to something like that? In my case, I didn't. I found that in order to be a cancer patient, you have to grow a very thick skin and totally ignore some people. Nevertheless, it still hurts to receive such remarks.

When I was first diagnosed, I called one of my neighbors who is a social worker to tell her the news. She was very calm during our conversation, and I thought, "She needs space to absorb what I am going through." Four months later, I still hadn't heard from her when I ran into her at the store.

"I've been meaning to call you," she began, "but quite frankly, I didn't know what to say to you, so I've said nothing. I mean, do you want to talk about it? Or, do we ignore the cancer and talk about something else? I just don't know what to do."

She wasn't the first person to say that, but she was the first person to question how we could make it better. So we got together, and I told her that if I wanted to talk about the cancer, I would. If I were feeling in a good mood and would prefer to talk about something else, so be it. The bottom line is *let the patient dictate the conversation*. Many people felt that they *had* to talk about the cancer and my future as a way of validating what I was going through. What they didn't realize was dying patients don't need validation. We just need conversation and support.

• • • • • • • • • • • • • • • • • •

Finding Humor Where You Can

The day after my diagnosis, my husband and I received a beautiful flower arrangement. As he placed the flowers on the bookcase, he gave me the card to open. The card was the standard florist card, the one that says, "With Deepest Sympathy" and has white lilies on the side. The note read: "You are in our thoughts and prayers." It was sent from close friends, and quite frankly, I was too dumbfounded to react; however, the feeling changed in a flash. "Just think, I've received my first sympathy card, and I'm not even dead yet!"

The point of this story is that when a person is dying, maintaining a sense of humor can be a valuable energizer. Who can argue that sending flowers at a time like this is a nice, thoughtful gesture, but receiving the accompanying card was truly upsetting ... until I began wondering when the fruit baskets were going to start arriving!

How To Talk To A Dying Person

- Ask simple, everyday questions. "How are you?" "What's new?" These questions might sound trivial, but dying people are no different than anyone else.
- Let the dying person dictate the conversation. The choice of discussing the illness lies with the person, not the friend.
- If the subject of illness or death comes up, silently pay very close attention and listen to what the person is saying. Too often, we feel we must make comments or try to contribute to the conversation. In reality, the dying person may need an avenue to vent feelings, worries and fears. Let the person talk without interruptions. Try to maintain eye contact.
- It is okay to show emotion to the dying person. Expressing your own fears and worries about the person's situation can create a bond between the two of you that serves as support and comfort.

•   •   •   •   •   •   •   •   •   •   •   •   •   •   •   •   •   •   •

Lessons Learned: Reactions

- Society denies death. By doing this, the needs of the dying patient are frequently ignored or misunderstood, resulting in unnecessary suffering.
- Society's fear of death is a by-product of the introduction of medical technology. Because ever-improving machines and equipment offer the opportunity to extend life beyond normal expectations, people are confused by false hopes and promises. Once again, this results in pointless suffering and grief.
- What doctors don't realize is that when a patient dies, it is not their failure. Rather, it is the individual's body that has failed!
- By openly discussing death with friends and health care providers, an atmosphere of acceptance and support can be generated to help the patient deal with impending demise. This open awareness allows everyone to honestly be involved in caring for the dying person.
- While society in general does not want to deal with death, individuals do. People are eager to talk about their own experiences with death as a way of trying to understand life's final end and the lessons to be learned from it.
- Dying people are just like everyone else. Do not feel scared to talk or interact with a dying person. Rather, comfort and support can be gained through social interaction at a time when the patient is facing the greatest challenges.

4

Thinking It Through

It is never too soon to begin planning, although often it is too late. Before things got more out of hand on the wild train ride through medicine, I decided to have a long talk with myself to map out what I wanted for my final days. My training and background taught me that it is best to have this kind of talk with yourself and loved ones long *before* illness strikes. And during my 12 years writing in the hospice and palliative care field, Joe and I did talk a little bit about "what if," usually when I was telling him about an anonymous patient I had met. But those talks were nothing like the ones we are forced to have now!

Like a pregnant woman who chooses how and where she wants her baby to be born, I knew that I had the ability and knowledge to carve out my death as I wanted, rather than leaving this important final step to the doctors and nurses. What it all boiled down to was what I, the patient, perceived to be "a good death." "The 'needs' of the dying patient are defined and thus filtered through the views of family and health care professionals," wrote the editors of the well-respected *British Medical Journal* in 2003. "The authority over dying must now be invested in patients. Patients' concepts of a good death should guide our efforts to make deaths better." [1]

What is "A Good Death"?

What makes a "good" or "bad" death? How does a person define this important factor in end-of-life care? According to the U.S. government's Institute of Medicine:[2]

"A decent or good death is one that is: free from avoidable distress and suffering for patients, families, and caregivers; in general accord with patients' and families' wishes; and reasonably consistent with clinical, cultural, and ethical standards.

. . . .

"A bad death, in turn, is characterized by needless suffering, dishonoring of patient or family wishes or values, and a sense among participants or observers that norms of decency have been offended. Bad deaths include those resulting from or accompanied by neglect, violence, or unwanted and senseless medical treatments."

From a dying person's perspective, I don't find these definitions very comforting. They are too generic and not specific enough to suit my individual needs. Reflecting on my fellow chemo patients who come from all different backgrounds and ethnicities, I'm not sure they would benefit from these definitions either.

Looking at death from different cultural and ethnic points of view yields a wide variety of definitions. For example, some people—usually deeply religious people—choose to suffer at the end and refuse pain medications. They see death as atonement for their sins in this life. Others want many family members and friends to surround them, praying and chanting, during their final moments. While some people may choose to have a serene and peaceful death, there are those who are willing to "fight to the end" and seek aggressive treatment up until the minute they die.

The choices are as individual as each of us; however, there are some common factors that are important for the majority to have a good death.[3] They include:

- Control of symptoms;
- Preparation for death;
- Opportunity for closure or "sense of completion" of life;
- Good relationship with health care professionals.

Despite these commonalities, there *cannot be one definitive explanation of "what is a good death."* It is a deeply personal and intimate decision that each of us must make at some point in our lives. What might suit my definition of "a good death" might not agree with anyone else's—this is the beauty of individuality and personal preference.

Why is defining "a good death" so important? Because if a person doesn't do this crucial retrospection, then who knows what will happen during the final days?

Few people would remember Henry Sullivan. He was a famous composer and musician in the 1930s and 1940s. In addition to writing what is commonly

• • • • • • • • • • • • • • • • • • • •

known as "the circus music," Hank was a prolific composer of Broadway tunes. At the height of his fame, he had four shows on Broadway at the same time, and he mingled in such celebrity crowds as Laurence Olivier, Richard Burton and Alec Guinness. To the public, he was a successful artist who "had it all." But to me, Hank was the closest thing I had to a grandfather. As a good friend of my grandmother's ("Big Laura"), Hank was always around for family get-togethers, birthday parties and holiday celebrations. Because both of my grandfathers died before I was born, Hank filled in this void in our family.

Hank fell on hard times when he was in his 60s. Mismanagement of money, bad health and few friends threw him into such a deep depression that he failed to take care of his health. As a result, Hank entered a nursing home in upstate New York where he lived anonymously for three years. At his death in 1965, he was alone in a dark room, without anyone to support him, and he died in considerable pain. Despite signing important Broadway contracts and other business papers, Hank had failed to fill out a living will or appoint a health care power of attorney, so no one knew what he wanted for his final time on this earth. Nor did anyone know where he wanted to be buried, so he ended up in a pauper's grave that no one can find.

Hank's story also highlights problems in end-of-life care that continue to exist 40 years later. Like Hank, many people are in nursing homes and hospitals during their final days, two places where finding "a good death" is challenging. According to the "Family Perspectives on End-of-Life Care at the Last Place of Care" study, published in 2004, inadequate pain management, little emotional support and poor communications from physicians occurred on a regular basis. In fact, poor pain management was 60 percent more likely to occur in a nursing home than in a private home where the patient was getting hospice care, and 20 percent of the patients in the nursing home said they weren't treated with respect.[4]

The point of this story is that "bad deaths" can happen to anyone, even the famous, wealthy and talented composers of the world. The only way to avoid this is to take control of your life and put your wishes in writing.

. . . .

Decision-Making: Healthy Versus Sick?

Having worked in the end-of-life field for several years, there have been many times that I have thought, "What would I do if I got sick?" When I was healthy, my answers were very black and white. "If I were diagnosed with cancer, of course I would have chemotherapy," I would say. "I would do whatever it takes to get well."

But as a diagnosed cancer patient, my answers fall into more gray areas. "I'll have this chemotherapy even if it means I'll lose my hair, vomit all the time and feel awful. But if it permanently damages my eyesight so that I go blind, then I'm not so sure I'll continue with it."

When I was healthy, I never thought about quality-of-life issues related to whatever illness I would contract. I just thought myopically about the disease and its cure. But all treatments for all diseases have side effects, and this is realized only when a person must go through the experience.

Few medical professionals see treatment and its side effects as a package deal. Rather, treatment and effects are separated out as two distinct and different entities. To the pros, talking about treatment and discussing side effects are two entirely separate conversations where one is showcased and the other ignored. As a result, when presented to the dying person, there is "no one big picture" to look at that would help in decision-making. Dying people need to know the gray areas of their illness. It is their right to information, which can empower them to make difficult decisions based on facts, not feelings.

Creating My Own Definition

I decided that because I was the person who was going to die, I had to find my own definition of what is "a good death" by *my* standards. How does a person make these kinds of decisions? In my case, I began by hypothesizing what my death will look like:

Where do I want to die (hospital, home or nursing home)? I want to die at home.

Who do I want with me at the time when I die? I want only my husband by my side when I take my final breath; however, I want someone in the house at the time that can provide emotional and practical support to my husband after my death.

• • • • • • • • • • • • • • • • • • • •

Are there any medical concerns that I want known? I do not want to die in pain.

Should certain medications be withheld from my care because of addiction or mortality concerns? My primary fear is dying in pain. I have no concerns regarding the use of pain medications. So, whatever it takes to keep me out of pain is all right with me.

Should certain medical procedures be withheld from my care at the end? I don't want to be kept alive by artificial means, such as feeding or breathing tubes and the like at the end.

Is there any situation where I would consider assisted suicide? No. Let nature and God guide the process.

How do I see my death? I want my death to be dignified, peaceful and comforting.

Have my wishes for burial been conveyed? Yes. My husband knows where I want to have my funeral and burial. We made the arrangements together.

Seizing Control

In the ever-changing medical arena, it is even more important that terminally ill people and their health care representatives become active advocates not only for health-related matters but for death-related issues as well. Most people don't realize that they can control their own death. They fail to recognize they are empowered to make choices, opt for treatment, and tend to final matters without input from the medical profession.

Through advance directives, a person (healthy or terminally ill) simply writes down his wishes and desires for his death and then appoints a health care representative to speak for him when he cannot. They are two of the most valuable documents that a person will ever have. Making wishes known, both orally and in written form, gives a person the power to govern his death.

• • • • • • • • • • • • • • • •

What are Advance Directives?

Advance Directives is a general term that applies to two types of legal documents:

- A *Living Will* allows a person to put in writing what medical treatments he or she wants at the end of life. For example, do you want a feeding tube? Cardiopulmonary resuscitation? Curative or comfort care? A Living Will should not be confused with a regular will, which allows the person to leave material possessions and assets to loved ones. A regular will is a separate document that does not impact medical care.
- A *Health Care Power of Attorney*, also known as a *Medical Power of Attorney*, allows a person to appoint someone to make medical decisions when that person no longer can act in his or her behalf.

Some doctors are now highlighting advance directives by including them in the introductory patient information kit, right behind medical and insurance information. This way there is something written down in case of emergency, and the wishes can be changed whenever the patient desires. Both documents can be easily obtained from doctor's offices, medical agencies and hospitals as well as downloaded from the Internet.

Many people store these documents in a safe deposit box, but completed copies should be given to personal physicians, to the hospital when the patient is admitted, and other copies can be kept at home and in the car in case of emergencies.

To be sure that the personal wishes of the dying person are followed, there must be a concerted effort to learn everything about the disease so that informed decisions can be made. Once the decisions regarding death are complete, the person should talk to family members and doctors beforehand about what is envisioned for the final days. Many people avoid talking about end of life because of their fears: suffering, pain, separation from loved ones and the unknown. These fears keep them from dealing with life's final lesson and make it harder to plan their lives as they wish. Not talking can also make it harder for those left behind. So the sooner this discussion occurs, the better for the patient, family members and medical professionals.

• •

Joe: The Business Side

Any serious illness often results in a tremendous volume of paperwork. To keep everything organized, Laura and I put the paperwork in a binder along with names, addresses and phone numbers of all physicians, notes we took at medical appointments, hospital discharge instructions, test results and reports from the home care nurse. We also kept a list of all medications, noting what they were for and the dosages. I kept a log of when all medications were administered, especially noting each dosage. This was very helpful when talking with the physicians and hospice nurse.

I put Laura's advance directives in the binder in the event paramedics had to be called to the house. We kept a magnetic calendar on the refrigerator to record medical appointments.

Medical expenses for a prolonged illness easily run into hundreds of thousands of dollars. Insurance coverage relieved a lot of my stress about the cost of Laura's care. Many of Laura's physicians filed claims directly with the company, which was very helpful in facilitating the process. Our insurance company's case manager assigned to Laura monitored her treatment and acted as a liaison with her health care providers and hospice. I reconciled medical bills with insurance coverage on a frequent basis.

Laura: The Importance of Patient Autonomy

Being a medical professional can be a double-edged sword when dealing with a dying patient. When a patient first presents with an illness, any doctor or nurse will jump right in to help that person deal with the problem. It is part of the humanitarian nature of medicine, and patients expect and demand such behavior.

But all too frequently, in the rush to help, the patient's autonomy—or ability to make decisions for herself—is lost or forgotten. Instead of seeing a person who has free will and judgment, many medical professionals tend to relate only to the disease, forming a kind of "relationship" with the disease, not the patient. This creates a gap in communication between the patient and the medical staff, one that the patient carries throughout the course of the disease. Focusing on the disease instead of the person results in the patient feeling a loss of control over her body and her life.

. . . .

Patients must feel as if they still have some control over their lives. Some might turn over control of their bodies to medical professionals yet want to control symbolic decisions. Others might wish to make all-important decisions regarding treatment while others might turn over such decision-making to their health care power of attorney. No matter which path the dying patient chooses, there is always an element of self-regulation and control.[5]

By not respecting a patient's autonomy, an antagonistic relationship is created between health care professionals and their patients. In addition, this loss impacts on the patient's inner self. For the patient, losing control is losing self-esteem and losing hope. Without these two elements, no patient can effectively deal with a disease or its many ramifications, including impending death.

In following the national Patients' Bill of Rights, medical professionals must give their patients a sense of control over their lives and their bodies at a time when everything else in the patient's life is chaotic.

Defining the Boundaries of Treatment

The approach used to define "a good death" can also be used towards setting limits on treatment. This is important because the choices made in treatment might impact on achieving a good death. A dying person may, for instance, choose to have treatment that requires hospitalization. What if the person dies in the hospital during one of these sessions? Does it conflict with his desire to die at home?

Frequently, doctors will prescribe aggressive curative treatment in an attempt to save the dying person's life. They put on blinders and go all out, drawing on all of the vast resources available in the medical arena without regard to the side effects of what they are prescribing. The dying person is left to deal with these symptoms.

As an example, I was born with growths over my eardrums, which made me considerably deaf. After months of radium treatments and surgery, I finally was able to have a limited level of hearing by the time I was six. In order to compensate for my lack of hearing, I relied upon my eyesight to absorb daily events and conversations.

This vignette is important because I learned that one of my chemo drugs for pancreatic cancer could impact and diminish my eyesight. This was not acceptable to me. My eyes are too important to me. If the drug were to diminish my sense of hearing, that would be acceptable because I'm used to having inferior auditory ability. But to take away my vision—probably the most important sense to me—would be far more upsetting. I told both Joe and my doctor that if my eyesight began to suffer because of the chemo, then I would stop the chemo.

While some of the issues related to end-of-life care haven't changed for years, new issues make decisions even more challenging. In particular, health care has changed so quickly that there are new medical technologies and treatments that can extend your life well beyond its natural course, if that is what you want.

But sometimes the treatment can be worse than the disease. That's what happened to my "chemo pal" Anne, a 67-year-old with breast cancer. She and I had been doing chemo together for four sessions and inasmuch as I knew my chemo for pancreatic cancer was rough, it became apparent that she couldn't tolerate her chemo regimen much longer.

"I just wanted to wish you luck," said Anne (cancer patients never say "goodbye"). "I'm here to get my records, and then I am going home. No more treatment for me!"

"But I thought your treatment was working," I said, incredulously. "What happened?"

"It's not a question of whether the treatment is working," she replied. "I'm just sick of being sick all the time. I have treatment on Tuesday and then feel awful for the rest of the week. The vomiting and nausea never seem to really go away. I don't have a favorite food anymore because everything tastes so bad. I can't even have my lovely little glass of wine anymore! By the time I start to feel a little bit better, it is time for another chemo session, and the routine begins all over again."

Her eyes began to fill with tears, and I took her hand. I didn't really know what to say, but I knew exactly how she felt. I had felt that way many times. In fact, it became a joke between Joe and me that every time I had chemo, there would be an awful moment when I would turn to him and say, "This is it. No

♦ ♦ ♦ ♦ ♦ ♦ ♦ ♦ ♦ ♦ ♦ ♦ ♦ ♦ ♦ ♦ ♦ ♦ ♦ ♦

more chemo! I can't take it anymore." But then I would show up for the next session, deluding myself that this time it might be better. That was never the case.

"Anne, you're choosing quality of life over quantity of time, and I admire you for that," I said. "Everyone has to do what is right for them, and if chemo is making you so miserable, then it is time to quit."

"I just want to be able to do the things that I want to do, not what chemo's side effects allow me to do. I want to die happy, and chemo won't allow that. But now, I can do what I want to do, and I've given this a great deal of thought," she said. "Guess what? I'm taking my children and grandchildren on a cruise off of Greece for 10 days. If that doesn't make me happy, then nothing will!"

Dying patients and family members must decide which symptoms they can deal with and which are unacceptable as a way of controlling the steps leading up to death. All people—terminally ill as well as healthy individuals—must be strong advocates for their care at the end of life. It is never too soon to begin planning, although often it is too late.

Lessons Learned: Patient's Wishes

- There is no one definitive explanation of "what is a good death." It is a deeply personal and intimate decision that each of us must make at some point in our lives.
- Find your own definition of "a good death."
- The best way to convey your final wishes is through a Living Will, which describes what you do and do not want in treatment. By appointing a health care power of attorney your chosen representative can speak on your behalf to ensure that your wishes are followed.
- Talk to your power of attorney, family members, close friends and medical professionals about your final wishes. This way, everyone is "working off the same page" in an attempt to honor your wishes.
- Sometimes the treatment can be worse than the disease.

5

The Medical Side of Dying

Oncologists are the "pit bulls" of the health care field. I say this affectionately because when you are a very sick patient, they are the ones who will pursue every course of treatment, examine every aspect of care, and push standard medical limits in order to find a cure and to save your life.

But when a person is diagnosed with cancer, the simple act of meeting the oncologist for the first time takes on a deeply spiritual and more profound meaning. This is the person who not only is going to run your life for a period of time, but who might oversee your death as well. Psychologically, this person's power over the patient is awesome, intimidating and terrifying.

So, it was no wonder that Joe and I showed up very early for our first appointment with Dr. Kenneth Miller, my oncologist. Both of us were nervous not only about what to expect from this visit, but also in dealing with the residual feelings of shock from the diagnosis. After all, Monday, I went to Dr. Meyer; Tuesday, I learned the diagnosis; and now Thursday, I am meeting my oncologist for the first time. Everything was happening too fast for us to absorb the true meaning of the events. This is a common reaction, it turns out, because patients, who should be preparing for the end of life, might not be able to process the information fast enough to keep pace with events or might remain in denial.[1]

For me, the stress of this first meeting affected my stomach, and I became very nauseous in the parking lot. I spent most of the time doubled over in the car, trying hard to calm myself down. In addition, I felt that my anxiety was out of control—I didn't want to be "here," I didn't want to be "there," I just wanted to be "someplace else" so that I didn't have to deal with my illness. Joe, too, was nervous, pacing around the parking lot and constantly looking at his watch. We both knew we were about to meet the future—one that was too painful to discuss.

· ·

But our feelings subsided when we approached Dr. Miller's office. Our appointment was at 9 a.m., and the office, which is a group practice of five oncologists, has a rule that it does not unlock the doors until 9 on the dot. Because we were a few minutes early, Joe and I joined the other patients in the hallway, some standing and others sitting.

I must admit that I had always thought of cancer patients in the office setting as being very somber, distant and depressed as a group. After all, the issues being faced are certainly profound and sobering. But to my surprise, what I found was quite the opposite: most are very open and friendly. They are quick to say, "Hello," even if they feel terrible, and while each person is depressed about his or her particular situation, there is a sense of community amongst cancer patients. *"We're all in this together"* is an underlying feeling that I sensed more than once when going to the doctor's office.

What I quickly learned was that when you have cancer, you join a very select club where everyone knows everyone else. Because we were "new to the club," all of the 10 patients who were standing in the hallway introduced themselves. One by one, they told us what kind of cancer they had, what their treatment was, and, most importantly to me at the time, what they thought of their doctor. I told them about my cancer and how we were still in a daze from what we were going through, and each member of the group said they went through the same thing.

"I still have those feelings," said one elderly man who had leukemia. "And it's been three years since my diagnosis! I still can't believe it is happening to me!"

By the time the doors opened, we felt as if we had been attending an informal cancer support group, which helped me to realize that I was not alone. It was one of those valuable "accidents" that taught me about the camaraderie of cancer as well as the importance of sharing the experience of illness. Those few minutes in the hallway gave both Joe and me the kind of tremendous comfort that only another cancer patient can give.

* * * * * * * * * * * * * * * * * * * *

Not All Cancers Are Alike

It seems that when I tell others about my cancer, everyone has a similar story. Either a parent, friend or even the individual has suffered through the experience of cancer. Sometimes it feels as if we are having a contest to see whose treatment and diagnosis is worse!

What few people realize is that each cancer is different. Not only are the tumor cells of each person distinctive, but also each treatment, diagnosis and prognosis for the future is unique. Each cancer is as individual as each person.

But when I mention my pancreatic cancer, friends and family members often equate it to more curable cancers, such as breast or prostate. In the beginning, it was hard to convince a dear friend like Kathy that her melanoma, which was surgically excised and required no further treatment, is totally different from my pancreatic problem. To many, cancer is cancer, regardless of location on or in the body, or survival rate for that type of cancer.

Unfortunately, my diagnosis of adenocarcinoma pancreatic cancer is considered to be one of the worst forms of the disease. As the fourth leading cause of cancer deaths in the United States, pancreatic cancer was set to kill 30,000 Americans in 2003 alone. This is out of the 30,700 who were diagnosed in that particular year. Only 700 patients would survive one year after diagnosis![2] Even more telling, only four percent of those with pancreatic cancer would be alive in five years.[3]

These statistics make the virulent and lethal natures of this type of cancer too clear. Worse yet, compared to other cancers, little research is being done to treat pancreatic cancer.

This is not to say that those with other cancers don't suffer from the same anxieties and pain as pancreatic cancer patients, but there is a greater reason for hope with other cancers. With pancreatic cancer, there is no hope in the traditional sense. Knowing that pancreatic cancer is incurable, I realize that people mean well by relating stories of "how I beat cancer." But instead of giving inspiration and hope, these stories frequently result in making the dying person feel the opposite: utter disheartenment and hopelessness.

• • • • • • • • • • • • • • • • • • •

Pancreatic Cancer

Dr. Miller spent a great deal of time going over my CAT scan with us. He told us that the pancreas lies deep within the abdomen, between the stomach and the spine, and this positioning makes it difficult to detect any abnormalities, such as a tumor. By the time a tumor is found, it is usually too late, and that is what happened in my case. The pancreas makes hormones, including insulin, to regulate blood-sugar levels, and it is responsible for the enzymes that are needed for digesting food.[4]

Dr. Miller told us that my relatively young age was a potential advantage because most people who are diagnosed with pancreatic cancer are between the ages of 60 and 80. While no one really knows what causes the disease, it is significant that both of my father's birth parents died at young ages of diabetes, a disease linked to the pancreas. Heredity, I learned from Dr. Miller, is a key factor in this disease because pancreatic cancer tends to run in families.

The pancreas is comprised of three parts: the head (the widest part), the middle section, and the tail. While most pancreatic tumors are located in the head, mine unfortunately occupied about one-third of the tail of the pancreas. Because the cancer had already metastasized to my liver and one lung, my diagnosis was *Stage IV* (the end stage), which precluded me from being considered for radiation or surgery. My only option, Dr. Miller explained, was chemotherapy.

But before any treatment could start, we had to find out more about the cancer growing in my body. The PET scan was scheduled first, with a biopsy set for the next day. This schedule only compounded my anxiety, and I began to feel overwhelmed and emotionally numb.

"As if the stress of finding out about the cancer wasn't enough, now I have to endure these tests," I thought to myself. *"What if they find something else wrong with me?"*

As a medical writer, I am used to the investigational part of an illness where all kinds of tests are run to determine what is truly going on in the patient's body—but not my body! I remember sitting with one woman in particular who had just found out that her seven-year-old daughter had a brain tumor. The surgeon had scheduled a battery of tests for the child who had never been sick a day in her life before this event.

* * * * * * * * * * * * * * * * * * *

"Everything will be okay," I told the mother. "The doctor is one of the finest in the country, and your daughter will be good as new in no time."

I never realized the impact of what I was saying. While I thought I was giving the mother hope and reassurance, I was, in fact, minimizing the daughter's illness. I had fallen back on platitudes and stock answers to comfort this woman, and it is no surprise to me that I failed in this mission. Now that I am the patient, I can see what the mother and child were up against, and my words dim in a different light.

The PET Scan

On July 11th, I showed up for the PET scan, full of dread and anxiety. Fortunately, I was surprised that the test wasn't too stressful. The worst part, it turned out, was the day before when I followed a specially designed diet that emphasized eating protein.

Upon my arrival, I was taken into a small examination room where the lab technician injected me with radioactive glucose. I just had to lie there for 45 minutes and not move so that the material could navigate through my body. Then I was placed on a special CAT scan machine that divided the body into eight segments. Each segment took several minutes to scan. The radioactive isotopes from the injection bound with the cancer cells to produce white circles on film indicating where cancer was located in my body.

In getting the results, Dr. Miller told us that the cancer had spread from my pancreas to my lungs and liver. In particular, my liver showed five "spots" or lesions, reflecting considerable damage. After I read the PET scan report, I questioned him about other areas in my body that had been highlighted. He said it was "nothing to worry about" and that chemo is systemic so all of my organs would benefit.

Once the PET scan was over, I had to steel myself for the next step—the biopsy. There is no way I can adequately describe my feelings at this point. Numb. Terrified. Overwhelmed. Desperate. These are just a few that came to mind. Just one week before, I thought I was a healthy woman with a minor health problem. Now I felt like I was a walking, talking and feeling blob of

• •

cancer. I was so demoralized and hopeless, thinking what was the point of going on with any medical procedures (and life too) because the cancer had spread so far.

I was also dumbfounded in realizing how far the cancer had advanced. How could it get this far, and I didn't know it?

How Misunderstandings Occur

Throughout the therapeutic relationship, many times the doctor/patient relationship can become easily compromised. A prime example is when I asked Dr. Miller about the "other" spots on my PET scan. He minimized their presence, leading me to think that they didn't really exist.

However, when I went back for my retesting two months later, I found out from the radiologist that the previous scan clearly showed that the cancer was indeed also in my bladder, colon, urethra and uterus. In fact, the film looked like a photo of a Dalmatian! While the cancer cells were fewer after chemotherapy treatments, they were there nevertheless.

From the doctor's point of view, the cells in those other organs weren't enough "to worry about." He wanted to concentrate on the organs that had the most cancer. But to me, the person who owns this body, my attitude was "if there is any cancer anywhere, I want to know about it. Even if there is one cell in my big toe, I want to know!"

While I don't feel that Dr. Miller lied to me, he certainly didn't tell me the truth either. He was looking at the overall grand picture while I was focusing on the minute details. Both of us were looking at the same picture with different glasses. But this difference in interpreting the facts can create mistrust between the doctor and patient, which can impact on all levels of the therapeutic relationship. What is important to the patient might be different than what is important to the doctor, but because it is the patient's life on the line, every effort should be made to fully inform the patient of the disease's presence and progress, even if the doctor thinks the information is trivial and unimportant in the grand scope of the illness.

• • • • • • • • • • • • • • • • • • • •

The Biopsy

The biopsy was scheduled for July 16th. When we arrived at the hospital the next day for the procedure, I didn't care what happened.

"With the cancer being in so many places, why even bother with the biopsy?" I thought. *"Why put myself through this hell? What was the point of trying to find out what kind of tumor it was? What difference would it make?"*

All I knew (and cared about) was that the tumor was big and aggressive and that the cancer was everywhere, growing faster with each passing minute. Naturally, I was becoming more terrified by the minute, and most of my energy was going into preventing the emotional paralysis that the cancer could cause.

When Dr. Miller and I first talked about the biopsy, he explained that they would put me on a CAT scan table and then insert a fine needle into my pancreas to get a sample. Seeing the look of panic on my face, Dr. Miller said that he thought it would be best if I were put to sleep for it, and I quickly agreed. The less I knew what was going on the better because my nerves were so frayed.

However, the hospital people had other ideas about this. In procedures like this, patients usually are given twilight-sleep sedation because it "makes recovery so much easier." I tried to explain to the scheduler that I already knew that there was a tumor; I was stressed beyond my capabilities and that general anesthesia was the only option I would consider. For her, however, there was no other option.

What I couldn't make the hospital scheduler understand was that within a one-week period, I learned I had terminal cancer, met my oncologist, had a PET scan, and was preparing for chemotherapy. That is a tremendous amount of stress for anyone to handle, especially within such a short period of time. The biopsy, I told her, was just another chunk of stress placed on my body, and I didn't think I had the emotional reserve to deal with the procedure.

"Hospital protocol says that you should have sedation, not anesthesia," she said, "and I have to follow the rules. You won't feel a thing. Nine a.m. okay with you?"

This is just one instance where the rules that apply to "healthy" people are also mandated for the terminally ill, regardless of their feelings or needs. While I understand the benefits of having an easier recovery from a surgical procedure

• •

for a healthy person, the chronic anxiety and overall fear that each dying person lives with on a daily basis changes the wisdom of applying such an approach on the terminally ill.

The guidelines and standard practices that cover the healthy person should not be applied to the terminally ill. Dying people have their own special needs that are frequently ignored or bypassed because the rigid health care system "doesn't do it that way." Until these needs are recognized and honored, dying people will continue to suffer in small, degrading ways.

What are the Medical Needs of the Dying Person?

- To be accepted as an *equal partner* in decision-making and future planning.
- To acknowledge that the *person has the ultimate control* over medical decisions.
- To be told the *whole truth* regarding treatment and its side effects so that the person can make intelligent and wise choices based on individual preferences and characteristics.
- To have *full knowledge regarding medications* available, including pain, antianxiety and antidepression alternatives.
- To have *psychological and emotional issues considered* when ordering treatment and testing. Tests, such as MRIs and CAT scans, are terrifying to patients. Health care professionals should make the time to "introduce" the patient to the technology so that answers can be given to worrisome questions. By having a "dress rehearsal," the patient will be calmer and less nervous, making the health care professional's job a lot easier.
- To *see the patient as a frightened and emotional human being* rather than as the host of a disease that must be conquered.

The only way that I won this fight with the hospital was by threatening to cancel the procedure altogether. In agreeing to the general anesthesia, the hospital person pushed me to the end of the schedule list. Instead of being taken at 8 a.m., I was placed in the 2 p.m. slot—a huge difference because I couldn't eat or drink anything that day. I felt as if I were being punished for asking for general anesthesia.

• • • • • • • • • • • • • • • • • • • •

My continued feelings of dismay quickly multiplied when the biopsy was delayed by unfortunate typical hospital delays. The first IV didn't work. Then they couldn't find the radiologist to do the procedure. When they did find him, all he kept saying was that he had done 18 procedures that day and they should hurry up prepping number 19 (me). Then the anesthesiologist had to be replaced because of an in-hospital meeting! By 4 p.m.— two hours late—I was hungry, thirsty, panicked and totally fed up with the situation.

I have always prided myself on being a good and agreeable patient. If the doctor or nurse asks me to do something, I do it because I know the importance of cooperation between medical staff and the patient; however, in this situation–for the first time in my life—I became a difficult, argumentative and uncooperative animal.

"What do you mean you can't find the anesthesiologist?" I asked. "This hospital isn't that big! If you can't find him, how do I know you can find my pancreas?"

The situation grew even tenser as the nurse doing vital signs told me that I had a fever.

"Have you been sick with a cold lately?" she calmly asked. "Any bad food?"

I gave her a blank stare.

Obviously this nurse did not know that I had a tumor, or she didn't know that malignant tumors can cause *tumor fever*. While this is normal, a tumor fever does indicate that something is seriously wrong with the patient. Even with this crucial bit of knowledge that implies cancer, the nursing staff continued to treat me as though I were a normal, healthy person present for a routine biopsy.

As if it weren't bad enough that I was acting like a screaming banshee, Joe, and a good friend of ours, Carolee, both of whom are normally polite and calm individuals, became equally anxious and ill tempered. Joe decided to try and find out what was causing the delay, and Carolee was trying to calm me down.

"Breathe," Carolee kept telling me over and over again. "Take another breath."

"I don't want to breathe. I've had enough," I said, beginning to flail my arms. "I want this IV taken out, and I want to go home ... NOW!" I began looking at the IV to see if I could take it out myself.

* * * * * * * * * * * * * * * * * * *

When the nurse came and refused my request, I became even more agitated and vocal.

"I am the patient," I stated matter-of-factly. "I have the control. I decide what happens to me, and right now, I want out of here. I don't trust you people to do the right procedure."

"You don't understand," the nurse told me. "Everyone who has cancer loses their control over their body. The doctors and nurses who are trying to help you are now running your disease and your life. You have no control, and you have no rights."

To reinforce what she was saying, she began to roll me down to the CAT scan room. Suddenly, she stopped the gurney, leaving me alone in the hallway, and ran back to her desk. She had forgotten to have me sign the consent form for the procedure.

"Just sign here so we can start," she said with a smile, pushing the pen in my hand.

You know how unforgettable moments can be found at the weirdest times? This was one of them. I first looked at the form, then I looked at her.

"If I don't sign this, you can't do the procedure, right?" I said.

"Yes. That's why you just have to sign right here," she said, trying to push my hand towards the dotted line.

"What if I refuse? Then you'd have to let me go home," and I began to smile slowly.

The look on her face made this precious moment absolutely delicious! She didn't say a word—the look of horror in her eyes said it all.

"Who has the power now?" I asked, with my hands sitting idly on my lap.

This little standoff lasted only about a minute but it gave me a tremendous sense of control over my life that I needed at this time ... even as I signed that stupid form!

Finally, in the CAT scan room, the anesthesiologist quickly put me to sleep. The first biopsy showed that my cancer was an *adenocarcinoma*, a very aggressive form of the disease, and it was decided to do a second biopsy for confirmation. Because he had to attend a departmental meeting, the anesthesiologist woke me up to wait for his replacement! *"Does the patient's health and well-being truly come first?"* I wondered.

* * * * * * * * * * * * * * * * * * * *

When the second anesthesiologist was finally located, I was put back to sleep so that my *mediport* (also known as a *portacath*) could be surgically implanted. The mediport is a vascular device that allows access to the venous system other than putting a needle directly into a vein. Surgically placed in the chest or underarm areas, it looks like an inch-and-a-half bump under the skin, and it provides open access to the patient's body for blood work and chemotherapy. By having a port, a patient doesn't have to "get stuck" with needles as much, and it lessens the trauma to veins that would ordinarily be used. Rumor has it that it is painless but from my experience, both the surgery to put the port in and the process by which to access it are very painful.

For some reason, it was decided to put my port on the underside of my left arm (rather than in my chest, which is the usual place) because "as a woman, I might like to wear summer dresses or short-sleeved blouses." This cosmetic reason still doesn't sit well with me, perhaps because every time I move my left arm, I can feel the port. Autonomy and control extends to physical control as well, as seen by this example. While I should have been consulted about where to place the port, it never occurred to me to ask.

During this time, Joe and Carolee were frantically pacing in the waiting room. Joe kept asking the nurse to please find out what was taking so long. She said she couldn't do that because she was "too busy." Finally, Joe saw the radiologist who explained that things were taking longer because of the change in anesthesiologists. I should be through, he said, by 6 p.m.

At 7:30 p.m. I finally made my entrance into the recovery room. Joe went up to the radiologist and told him, "For Christmas, I'm going to buy you a watch because you can't tell time." Even though I was extremely groggy from being put to sleep twice, the radiologist came to my bedside and began talking to me.

"You have a long and difficult road ahead of you," he told me. "Pancreatic cancer is one of the nastiest cancers, and you have to be strong and keep that fighting spirit up. You will be in my thoughts and prayers." With that, he abruptly turned and left.

The only reason I know he said this is because Joe and Carolee told me. I, of course, was still under the effects of the anesthesia so I don't remember even seeing him. While I'm sure he was well intentioned, I think the radiologist was

· · · · · · · · · · · · · · · · · ·

giving his "speech" to make himself—not me—feel better. Once again, a total lack of regard for the patient's state of mind. Everything in this scenario was for the benefit of the providers, not the patient.

At no time during this episode were my feelings taken into consideration. After all, I was "Procedure 19" that day!

In 1990, the Institute of Medicine (IOM) focused its sights on care for terminally ill patients and found "evidence of quality problems in end-of-life care."[5] Among the problems were:

- Overuse of care, such as unwanted treatments or hospitalizations and diagnostic tests that will not improve patient care but cause physical and emotional distress.
- Underuse of care, including failure to assess and treat pain, late referral for hospice care and premature hospital discharge.
- Poor technical performance, such as errors in surgical technique; and
- Poor interpersonal performance, including inept communication of difficult news.

As seen in my experience with the biopsy, the needs and rights of this dying patient were abused, and the concerns of the caregivers were ignored. Even though the Institute of Medicine acknowledged these problems in 1990, my experiences have shown that little has changed. And I can probably find "Procedures 1–18" who were at the hospital that day who feel the same way!

◆ ◆ ◆ ◆ ◆ ◆ ◆ ◆ ◆ ◆ ◆ ◆ ◆ ◆ ◆ ◆ ◆ ◆

6

Treatment

In the old days, when people learned they had cancer, there were no options. You just had the disease and then died from it. But since the 1950s when modern medicine was introduced, the fate of a cancer patient (and the face of the health care field) has changed radically. A patient can have the cancer carved out of the affected area by a highly skilled doctor using highly sophisticated technology (surgery), or the diseased tissue can be devastated by high-powered rays (radiation). In addition, potent (and potentially lethal) drugs kill both the cancer and healthy cells (chemotherapy). Each or all of these treatments have the power to heal or control the disease and its symptoms.

Chemotherapy

Because my cancer had *metastasized* (spread to other organs), my only hope for treatment lay with chemotherapy. Now I was facing potent and toxic drugs being infused into my body in an attempt to gain control over the cancer. Dr. Miller made it very clear that these drugs would not "cure" my cancer because it was so advanced. They would, however, hopefully help me buy additional precious time.

Having done a lot of work at Johns Hopkins, Dr. Miller was aware of the most cutting edge treatment, and he suggested that I take what they call *G-FLIP*. This "kitchen-sink" combination of five potent drugs (Cis-Platin, Gemzar, Leucovorin, Fluorouracil [5-FU] and Camptosar) is infused continuously over a 48-hour period. After that, there is nothing for two weeks until the process is repeated.

"This protocol has been most promising," said Dr. Miller. "Since we can't cure your cancer, we are going to try to control it."

• • • • • • • • • • • • • • • • • •

While I knew that chemo was going to be rough—both physically and emotionally—I wasn't prepared for exactly how bad it was going to be. While nausea and diarrhea might result from any of these drugs, each has its own set of side effects. Cis-Platin, for example, might cause nerve damage, hearing loss, kidney damage and bone marrow depression. Fluorouracil (also known as 5-FU) might cause hair loss, mouth sores, skin pigmentation and uncoordination. Gemzar might damage my liver and cause abdominal pain. Leucovorin might cause rashes or itching. And even though these drugs were administered during a 48-hour period, I felt miserable for the entire two weeks afterward.

Despite these potential side effects, I didn't feel as if I had an option. I also had to keep in mind that it was my choice to have chemo, not that it was being "forced" on me. I vowed to myself that I would not allow chemo to be used well beyond its benefit period. Too often, chemo is continued until close to death, which can take away from precious quality time for the dying patient and family members. My feeling was, *"I'm going to feel bad enough from the cancer—why compound it with feeling awful from the drugs?"*

This commitment to cure can sometimes hurt the patient when the effort has gone on too long. Dr. Sherwin Nuland in his book, *How We Die,* points out that part of this commitment comes from a "determined cockiness" that doctors acquire as a result of successful cancer treatments. "If this treatment can cure one patient, it will cure all of them" is a typical medical reaction that fails to take into account the nature of the disease and the individual characteristics of the patient. As a result, "treatment must be pursued until futility can be proven, or at least proven to the satisfaction of the physician."[1] As with most issues in the end-of-life field, the question must be asked: What about the dying patient? As Nuland says, "Doing more is likely to serve the doctor's needs rather than the patient's."[2]

Several studies have shown that the use of chemo in particular continues well beyond positive impact for dying patients. Calling it the "overuse of chemotherapy at the end of life," Dr. Ezekiel Emanuel found that 41 percent of dying patients received chemo in the last year of life. More frightening, 33 percent received it in the last six months of life and one in four patients underwent chemotherapy in the final three months of life.[3]

. . . .

These findings made me realize that I didn't want to be among the final two groups, so Joe and I began to make a personal plan of what my criteria were for stopping chemo. Would I stop chemo if it caused me to go blind? Deaf? Damaged my immune system so badly that I couldn't see any family members or friends? Physically destroyed my body? *The bottom line for me was that if the chemo hurt me more than helped me, then I would quit.* Examples I gave Joe included destroying too many of my blood cells, governing my life so that I would lose control, and interfering with the things I want to do. In addition, my eyesight has always been important to me, and I realized that I would choose my sight over the chemo, if the situation arose.

One Final Taste of the Real World

By the time chemo was to start, I felt that I had no control over what was going to happen. This didn't last long! The day before chemo was scheduled to begin, our house lost all power, including air conditioning for the 90-degree heat. Compounding this was the fact that one of Joe's cousins, Karen, had come for a visit. We thought she could take my mind off what was going to happen the next day. But with the power outage, Joe and I were faced with checking into a hotel for the night. We all agreed that I had to be well rested for treatment. Karen and my father-in-law gamely decided to stay at the house with our dog, Gracie.

I don't know if it was the stress of losing our electricity or that this happened during the visit of one of my favorite people or if I was nervous about chemotherapy, but as soon as Joe and I got into the hotel room, I began vomiting all over the room. This went on for over an hour.

I mentioned this to Dr. Miller the next day before I was to begin treatment (quite frankly, I was hoping he would delay chemo because I had the stomach flu), and he said that what I experienced was *anticipatory vomiting*. Identified more than 90 years ago by the Russian physiologist Pavlov, anticipatory nausea and vomiting (ANV) is a common behavior among cancer patients. It is estimated that up to 50 percent of all people receiving treatment experience some nausea or vomiting *before*, not after, they received chemotherapy. The biggest threat that ANV poses is that this psychological behavior can become

• • • • • • • • • • • • • • • • • • •

permanent, if not treated. If that happens, chemotherapy might have to be reduced, or controlling the nausea and vomiting might be more difficult.[4] I didn't know any of this when I showed up for my first chemotherapy session at Montgomery General Hospital in Olney, Maryland.

The Beginning of a New Life

To a dying patient, any treatment for disease is an awesome and God-blessed savior ... and it is a truly frightening and perilous monster! So when we checked into the hospital at 9 a.m. as scheduled, it was no wonder that both Joe and I were very anxious and jittery. We were apprehensive because even though we knew what drugs would be used and what side effects might occur, the great unknown was how my body would react to them. That is the one variable in health care that no one can predict. It is for this reason that it is standard practice to admit a newly diagnosed cancer patient to the hospital for the first chemotherapy session. However, there was a comforting yet tense aspect to this: for the first part of the chemo, I was going to be in a room right next door to the Intensive Care Unit. As Jackie, the unit nurse, told me, if anything happened, the doctors and nurses could take care of me quickly. I would be in this room for the next six hours so she could closely monitor me as I received the first three drugs. After that, I would be transferred to a room in the hospital where I would spend the rest of the two days.

As each drug was started, Jackie told me which one it was and how long it would run. I find this kind of knowledge very comforting because it gives me a sense of control—I can account for what will be happening to my body during the next 50, 60 or 75 minutes!

Just sitting in one place for hours on end can be very boring, and so I started to doze. I mention this because the next thing I remember, it is Sunday and I have been out of the hospital for 24 hours.

"Maybe this is my reaction to the drugs," I thought hopefully. *"Chemo may not be so bad after all."*

Because of my memory loss, I didn't know about the horrible time I had with nausea and vomiting during the two days. Joe and Dad said I kept the nurses very busy. I also didn't remember my roommate; Joe said we became very good friends. I didn't remember one thing from the two days that I was there.

• •

I found out later that because I was so nervous and anxious in the beginning, I had been given Ativan, the potent antianxiety drug, throughout my hospital stay. This was Dr. Miller's answer to my anticipatory vomiting, and it worked. I haven't experienced ANV since that first session. But no wonder I couldn't remember anything!

It took me about three days to begin feeling like myself. The most pronounced side effect was uncoordination resulting from the 5-FU. I looked like a person with Parkinson's disease—trembling, unsteady on my feet, unable to hold a glass or fork, and unable to go up and down the stairs on my own. This was frightening until we were told that these side effects were to be expected.

Side Effects: What You Don't Know Can Hurt You

There seems to be this unwritten rule in the healthcare system that patients should not know about what side effects a drug might cause until it is too late. "We don't want to panic the patient by telling him or her what might happen," one nurse told me. "Everyone has a different reaction, and if the patients were to know about possible side effects, it would make them more frightened and uneasy."

What the health care system doesn't understand is that keeping the patient in the dark regarding potential side effects creates more fear and anxiety. It is unfair to the patient to withhold or gloss over important information such as side effects. In my case, Dr. Miller gave me a printout of my drugs with "potential" side effects. Joe and I never discussed them or even addressed what we should do if any became apparent. Do we call the doctor immediately? Do we go to the hospital? These are just a few of the questions a patient has when faced with the unknown. Because we never talked about the side effects of any of the drugs that I was given, whenever a side effect appeared, such as tremors, we panicked.

Dying patients are more resilient and resourceful than the health care system gives them credit. Instead of waiting for side effects to appear and then dealing with them, patients and family members should be told from the very beginning what might happen. By doing so, patients won't panic at every little change and will feel more in control over the disease and their own lives.

* * * * * * * * * * * * * * * * * * *

In addition, the nausea continued to be a problem. Eating a grape, for example, sent me into a violent vomiting attack in the kitchen, and a sip of water that was too cold caused a similar attack in the bedroom. I quickly learned that if I coughed, I would also throw up. According to one of the nurses, the muscles that govern coughing and vomiting use the same body mechanisms. I learned to stifle a cough at all costs, and I invested heavily in Robitussin.

Because of the nausea, I lost 12 pounds with the first chemo, and eating was becoming a major challenge. Because the pancreas is located between the stomach and the spine, my body was vulnerable to digestive and eating problems. While most chemo patients have trouble eating due to the treatment regimen, the problem is compounded for pancreatic patients because of the location of the pancreas. One bite and my stomach would expand with gas, leaving me to feel bloated and full. Like all cancer patients, because of chemo's effects on taste and smell, none of my favorite foods were enticing. Poor Joe and Dad spent days trying to get me to eat, and it became a cause for celebration if I swallowed only four spoonfuls of chicken soup.

Throughout history, food has always been a symbol of nurturing and health, and my two Italian men were becoming more concerned as each foodless day went by. This was turned around when I realized that if I didn't eat, the subject of a feeding tube would be brought up and pushed on me. Through my writing work in the end-of-life field and due to my hospice experience as a volunteer caregiver, I learned of both the benefits and detriments of feeding tubes. While they do provide nourishment to patients who are, for example, in a coma, the site of the feeding tube can frequently become infected, causing additional suffering and discomfort. In addition, in a patient like me who is dying, a feeding tube holds the possibility of extending my life beyond what God and nature decree. So the argument becomes quantity versus quality of life. I want my final days to be rich with love, connectedness and peace rather than medically tussling with a tube that might require surgery to correct a defect or antibiotics to fight an infection.

So, I decided to meet Joe and Dad halfway on food issues. Gradually, we learned what my chemo-influenced taste buds liked and didn't like, and I began to eat more. And it is not just the taste and smell of food that is important. The *texture* too is crucial in enjoying food. For example, when I was healthy, I used to eat chicken four days a week. But during my first chemo, I put a small

* * * * * * * * * * * * * * * * * * *

piece of roasted chicken in my mouth and was totally revolted by its texture. The taste and smell had nothing to do with it. I cannot eat chicken because of this.

In addition, some foods are totally inappropriate to serve. For example, whenever I was in the hospital for chemo, I would spend a large part of the day (and night) vomiting. Yet it never failed that the hospital served a dinner that included rice with gravy. Perhaps it is only the dying person who would make the visual connection between vomit and rice and gravy, but as soon as the tray was put in front of me, I had to turn my head and move it away. Whether food is brought from home or supplied by the hospital's dietary staff, special consideration should be given to cancer patients who are going through chemo. Providing a special meal that didn't include anything to remind the person of the side effects of treatment would be better tolerated and certainly welcome.

Joe: Milkshake Dates

Meals sometimes became a challenge for Laura. Because of the chemo and the medications, her tastes were constantly changing. Foods that she could tolerate one day were distasteful the next. It wasn't a commentary on my cooking. I quickly learned to have backup food on hand. Laura seemed to always tolerate several foods, and I made sure these items were continually available. She would have small meals during the course of the day to make sure that she was eating enough. We also turned her dietary challenges into a special time by having "milkshake dates." At an agreed-upon time, I would make milkshakes, and we would sit and talk.

Laura: Looking for the Good

I found a "good" benefit in my diagnosis. For 30 years, I thought I had a bad gallbladder. Rather than have gallbladder surgery, I followed a strict low-fat diet, which meant I had to give up a lot of my favorite foods. Knowing that my gallbladder is fine, I am able to eat anything I want—Fritos, chocolate, ice cream and red meat. Joe says that I'm like a child wanting one of everything, and it gives me great pleasure to eat something I haven't had in years.

◆ ◆ ◆ ◆ ◆ ◆ ◆ ◆ ◆ ◆ ◆ ◆ ◆ ◆ ◆ ◆ ◆ ◆

The point of this is that happiness can be found, even at the darkest of times. Encourage the dying person to find his or her own small bits of happiness, no matter how stupid or inane it might appear. Anything that puts a smile on the face is worthwhile. Five minutes of pleasure can go a long way for a dying person!

The second round of chemotherapy was much easier, due in part to the fact that I wasn't full of Ativan. And being able to be aware of every aspect of chemo gave me a tremendous education. I learned which drugs I could easily handle and which ones were difficult. Camptosar, for example, affected my vision and speech and gave me tremendous headaches. The most frightening for me was Cis-Platin. As soon as the drug was introduced into my body, I could feel it working its way through my spine's bone marrow. This caused a certain amount of sharp pain—like needles being pushed through my spinal column—but, thankfully, it did not last long enough to require pain medication. Usually, the pain subsided after 30 minutes, and I considered it to be a small price to pay for living longer.

Hair Loss

I've never thought of myself as being a vain person. Yes, I wear a little makeup and try to look nice, but my attitude has always been, it is what is underneath that counts.

But for the past two days, I've been acting like a beauty queen before the pageant! All because my hair is falling out. It started gradually, a couple of strands after the first chemotherapy session, but now it is coming out in huge handfuls. It has gotten to the point where I don't want to wash my hair or even blow-dry it, which only scatters the strands over a larger area. Every time I touch my hair, I'm disgusted and upset. I keep telling myself "it'll grow back" and "it is a small price to pay to live longer." But in reality, I tell myself these are platitudes that just don't work. Losing my hair is not just a painful reminder of my illness. It represents losing a part of me of which I am familiar and proud. I don't know how I'm going to deal with the "new" bald me.

In an effort to gain control over this situation, I told Joe and Dad that I was going to get a buzz cut. Why wait for the inevitable to happen? Just one quick—and painful—visit to Diane, my hairdresser, and the beauty pageant is over.

• • • • • • • • • • • • • • • • • • •

Knowing how painful all of this was for me, Joe came home from work suddenly the next day and announced that we were going to buy a wig. I was surprised that he was more comfortable than me in a specialized women's shop! "Look at this one. It looks like you," he kept saying. Meanwhile, I just sat quietly in the fitting chair being resistant to every suggestion and not even looking around at all of the choices. Finally, he and the saleswoman settled on one wig and put it on me. "What do you think?" asked Joe. It is hard to describe the feelings a person goes through at a time like this. Yes, the wig was my color and style. Yes, it was as close to a perfect match as possible. But ... it wasn't me!

Our next stop was the hairdresser. As Joe was getting his hair cut, Diane took me into a back room where I had privacy, and she worked as fast as possible. I tried to wait for Joe before I saw my new "do," but my curiosity took over. It was such a shock to see myself without my hair. After all, it has been 51 years since the last time I was bald! I broke down, crying. "Do you think Joe will still love me looking like this?" I asked Diane. She opened the door, and Joe walked in. "What do you think?" she replied, as Joe walked over to give me a big hug. "I didn't marry your hair," he said. "I love you more now than ever."

When a person is dying, the element of control becomes very important. That is why I chose to cut my hair before it all fell out. It gave me that sense of self-empowerment. The disease dictates one course of action and the doctors steer toward another. The patient is left in the middle with little grounding or strength. Sometimes I feel as if the only thing I have left is me, but with losing my hair, even that—me—is eroding each day.

On the surface, losing hair is a trivial nuisance. But for the dying person, it takes on a much deeper and profound meaning. Unlike an actress who shaves her head for a role, a dying patient doesn't know when—or if—the hair will ever grow back. It is always in the back of the patient's mind that there might not be enough time.

It isn't just hair that has this kind of impact on the person. It is anything physical, such as nails or skin. Patients need help in redefining this physical body in ways they can accept. I've known too many dying patients who "didn't care" how they looked. These feelings are just part of the deep, painful depression

• • • • • • • • • • • • • • • • • •

that a dying person feels. I can still remember when I looked great, when my auburn hair was thick and shiny, when my skin was smooth, and my eyes sparkled. Now I look like a concentration-camp victim who is next in line for the gas chamber. But once I got over the initial shock, I adopted a new philosophy—this is me. Accept me as I am. It really is what is underneath that is important!

Bringing Chemotherapy Home

When I was finished with the second round of chemo, Dr. Miller approached me with the idea of doing chemotherapy at home. The plan would be that I would go to his office for the infusion of the "heavy duty" drugs and then go home and have 5-FU administered slowly by a pump. A home care nurse would hook me up and Joe would have to unhook, clean and flush out the catheter at the end.

The only problem with this scenario, I told Dr. Miller, was that it put the burden of my care on Joe who is phobic about anything medical or needle-related. I felt that Joe had enough stress in his life, he (and I) didn't need anymore, so I fought doing chemo at home.

But Dr. Miller insisted. "You'll be so much more comfortable at home," he said. This discussion went back and forth for two weeks. Finally, in exasperation, I asked him why he was pushing so hard. Was it because of insurance and financial reasons? After all, I knew that each chemo session in the hospital cost $5,000.

"It has nothing to do with money," he said. "You have such little time left. Why spend it in the hospital?"

Once I got my breath back from this remark, I realized what Dr. Miller was really saying. Every minute for me was precious, and I decided that I should be spending my time in my home with my family. Joe and I talked it over, and we decided to try it. As the nurses explained, there was nothing he could do to hurt me, and if all else failed, he could always take me to the hospital to finish the infusion.

· · · · · · · · · · · · · · · · · ·

So when the third round of chemo came along, I went to Dr. Miller's office in the morning to begin the three-drug infusion. At the end of the four hours, with me looking like a Parkinson's patient because of the 5-FU, Joe brought me home where Patty, my home care nurse was waiting. She taught Joe and me how to connect and disconnect the catheter. This was a particular challenge for me because the effects of *chemo brain* had already set in. Chemo brain occurs when the drugs interact with the brain's function due to the fact that the drugs were killing off some of the patient's brain cells.

It is kind of like a chemically induced Alzheimer's disease where the patient suffers from short-term memory loss, mental confusion, and decreased mental ability. Everything Patty taught us about the catheter had to be written down for me, and I felt like such a child.

Because Joe was so hesitant about the medical procedures, Patty and I decided to present this challenge to him in terms of solving a mechanical problem, not a medical problem. This approach lessened his anxiety because Joe, like most men, loves "toys." He quickly learned how to unhook the catheter, prepare and flush both saline and heparin syringes, and clamp off the catheter for tomorrow's chemo session. In his mind, he might as well be changing the oil on my car! And it worked!

Like all men who love gadgets, Joe was particularly intrigued by the pump, which infused the drug. Small and compact, the pump had nine buttons, each one carrying a designated duty. One tells you how much time is left during this chemo session. Another tells you the rate of the infusion. If I had been more mentally cognizant of what was going on, I would have agreed with Joe that the pump was "neat."

But my mind was cloudy due to the drugs, and the last thing I wanted Joe to do was play with the pump while I was hooked up. He wanted to try pushing every button, and I kept saying "No." Finally, he exploded in anger. "You won't let me do anything to make my job easier!" This went on for the full eight hours of the drip! I thought this was ironic because Dr. Miller wanted us to do chemo at home to foster more intimacy and love. Instead, it led to our first disagreement since my diagnosis! We resolved this dilemma by letting him play with the pump once I was disconnected and out of the room.

7

Key Medical Issues

Have you ever been so worried about something that you think you will lose your mind or do something rash to escape the problem? That is what terminally ill people face every moment of every day—an anxiety that reflects absolute terror and fear.

Anxiety: The Most Misunderstood Element in End-of-Life Care

Despite its commonality, anxiety in the dying person is rarely talked about or, even worse, understood. This came to light when I went to Georgetown University's Lombardi Cancer Center for a second opinion. A very nice resident came in to do the initial intake assessment and after completing the physical and neurological exam, he asked me a series of questions. "Are you in any pain?" "How is your eating?" "How bad is your depression?" Answers in hand, he said he was off to report his findings to the doctor. I stopped him.

"You asked about my depression but didn't ask about my anxiety. Why?"

"They're the same thing, so I didn't want to ask a question twice," he said.

Depression and anxiety are NOT the same thing! In many ways, they are totally opposite. While depression is widely defined and treated, anxiety is often mislabeled or ignored. The general definition of *anxiety* is "a universal and adaptive response to a threat," and mental health experts consider the onset of anxiety during a physical illness to be normal and short-lived.[1] However, when applied to the psychological needs of individuals who are dying, this sense of anxiety is heightened beyond accepted expectations and, therefore, deserves a full examination.

I am terrified of flying. Even though I am the daughter of an airline captain, I cannot get comfortable sitting in a heavy box 35,000 feet above the ground. One of the last times I flew was in 1972 when my mother and I, age 22, were

• • • • • • • • • • • • • • • • • • •

going from Madrid to London. As soon as I saw the plane, I "knew" it was going to crash. My mother, who was used to my behavior, took me to the airport bar where I had a glass of wine to calm down. Then I had another glass and yet still a third. By the time we were ready to board, I was beyond my alcohol limit, yet my mind was amazingly clear ... and I was still terrified! It seemed as though no amount of alcohol could take away my fear. I even drew blood from my mother's arm when we hit a bad air pocket. It was only when the plane landed that my anxiety stopped ... and the effects of the alcohol hit!

The point of this story is that anxiety supercedes every other emotion and feeling inside a person. This fear and stress, linked to each individual's survival instinct, is strong enough to prevent any chemical substance from being metabolized normally. Only when the source of my fear was gone did I return to normal.

Anxiety would have done anything to make me avoid the source of my fear. Depression, on the other hand, would have calmly led me on the plane in the hopes that it would crash to end my misery.

When a diagnosis of terminal illness is presented to a patient, there isn't enough time to become depressed. Instead, anxiety might be the first emotion felt and the one that dominates the individual's mental well-being. More people report they are anxious rather than depressed. According to the *American Journal of Nursing*, the prevalence of anxiety among people with cancer or AIDS has been reported as high as 39 percent as compared to 25 percent who experience depression.[2]

Once again, *the standard rules of health care must be adapted to the needs of the terminally ill.* While anxiety and panic attacks are manifestations of psychological issues in the healthy person, the same diagnosis does not apply to the terminally ill person. For anyone who is facing death, anxiety and panic are related to the person's confrontation with mortality. Rather than being psychiatric in nature, anxiety is part of the individual's profound biological, emotional, psychological and spiritual makeup that must be resolved in order to have "a good death." Unlike everyday events, which might cause a person to experience panic, there is no escaping the shadow of death once a diagnosis has been made. Whether apparent or not, death is always on the terminally ill patient's mind.

· · · · · · · · · · · · · · · · · · · ·

Depression evolves over a period of time; however, it only takes one second to become anxious. Even in shock and denial, the patient might exhibit physical symptoms, such as feelings of terror, rapid heartbeat, dizziness, muscle tension or shaking in addition to panic attacks. After a period of time, this anxiety leads to clinical depression, which is characteristic in end-of-life care.

For many patients who are imminently facing death, the greater concern is anxiety, not depression, because anxiety is highly correlated with unrelieved pain, as well as, emotional factors such as fear and family members' reactions.[3]

As the disease progresses, these factors become more prominent as death nears. This is why some people might become nervous and agitated, and can't sleep in their final days.

Treatment professionals should never undermine the depth of these emotions. Medications, such as Ativan and Xanax, should be made available to any dying person *from the moment of diagnosis* so the person is better equipped to deal with the formidable and frightening challenges to come. They should be viewed as "pain medications" for the soul.

In addition, the patient might benefit from alternative methods such as meditation or deep breathing, counseling or, as cited in the *Handbook for Mortals: Guidance for People Facing Serious Illness*, by "channeling your worry into productive endeavors."[4]

Depression

Joe and I call them "reality moments." It is when all of a sudden one of us starts crying for no obvious reason. Sometimes we cry together, but more often than not, we each do it alone and in the privacy of our own thoughts and feelings. These crying sessions usually happen around the time of chemo—a couple of days before, a week after—but these jags have also been known to happen spontaneously at no specific time. Our reality moments didn't begin until about one month after my diagnosis when the truth of our situation began to really hit us, and both of us admitted to being depressed.

When a person is first diagnosed, there is no time to be depressed (or to really "feel" anything). Doctor visits, PET scans, CAT scans, blood work and other medical procedures take up a lot of time and energy, both physical and psychic energy. While anxiety is running rampant during this shock period, depression really doesn't have a chance to set in. As one cancer patient told me during chemo, "I was too overwhelmed in the beginning to allow myself to get depressed. I was fighting too hard to find ways to live."

But once the routine of treatment and daily challenges gets under way, the dying person has a chance to sit back and take stock of the situation. This is when depression occurs.

It is only natural and human to get depressed when a person finds out that death is right around the corner. If someone is given unhappy news of any sort, being sad and depressed are normal and healthy responses.[5]

However, for the dying person who must process so many life facets on different emotional and psychological levels, depression can be overwhelming. Most people think that dying people are depressed solely because they are facing the end of their lives. That isn't true. It is so much more than that. Many symptoms generally associated with depression, including fatigue, failure to concentrate, weight changes and sleep changes, aren't good indicators of depression in people who are dying because the symptoms might be caused by the illness or its treatments.[6] Other signs of depression include diminished pleasure or interest in activities, agitation or slowing, inappropriate guilt, poor concentration, and recurrent thoughts of death or suicide.[7]

"Clinical depression is not normal," notes Dr. Ira Byock in his book *Dying Well*, "and simple support will not suffice ... while disability, discomfort, and a dismal prognosis can contribute to clinical depression, a person's susceptibility might have less to do with the immediate situation than with biology, heredity, temperament, and lifelong self-image and ways of relating to others."[8] Therefore, the person's personality and background play a huge role in how he or she will emotionally deal with impending death.

Because between 15- to 25-percent of cancer patients experience depression[9], it is important for dying people to be evaluated and assessed for this condition. Often, asking the simple question "Are you depressed?" can successfully screen for depression in end-of-life care.[10] Once identified, there are a number of interventions that can offer tremendous help to the person as well as to family members: antidepressant therapy, psychotherapy, counseling and support groups.

But psychotherapy can be detrimental to the dying patient if it is misguided or inappropriate. For example, Joe and I were referred by Dr. Miller to meet

• • • • • • • • • • • • • • • • • • • •

with his staff therapist, and the first couple of sessions covered the basic groundwork of our situation. Both Joe and I thought that things were going well with the therapy until we had a discussion that was upsetting and, in a way, very confusing.

The therapist told me that I was thinking of myself too much as a dying person, not as a living person.

"You are being too negative," she said. "You're still a living human being and should be thinking that way. Plan future events and activities. Get involved in life in an active way."

I reminded her that I was the one with pancreatic cancer that has already spread to two other major organs in my body. From all medical sources, my prognosis was pretty grim. I told her that I thought I was being realistic about my condition and my future.

Then she mentioned Elizabeth Kübler-Ross's five stages of dying (denial, anger, bargaining, depression and acceptance), and her contention was that I should be in the denial stage because I had received my diagnosis less than a month before.

"Everyone goes through the stages differently," I said. "You can't put a timeline on them. Besides, it is easy for me to accept my diagnosis. I've seen the CAT scan films. I've read the radiology reports and blood work printouts. How can I deny what the results are when my own eyes have seen the evidence?"

This discussion went on for the entire session, and when we walked out of her office, we had questions about the benefit of future sessions. My attitude was that the discussion should be about my feelings and how to cope with them, not her perception of how I should be thinking. But for a dying patient, there isn't enough time to make major attitudinal changes or to question the therapist.

Prescribing the Unknown

It has happened to me more than once that a doctor has prescribed a procedure, treatment or medication without knowing anything about it. The most recent case of this oversight was when my nerve block was ordered to alleviate my pain.

* * * * * * * * * * * * * * * * * * * *

I asked one of the nurses in Dr. Miller's office about the procedure. Was it painful? What were the side effects? How long would it take me to recuperate? All she said to me was, "I don't know. Ask Dr. Miller." Oncologists are very busy people, and it isn't always easy to just pop into the office to ask a simple question. When I finally got hold of him, I asked him the same questions and his reply was that the surgeon would be the best qualified to answer my questions.

It would be extremely beneficial to a patient if someone in the office were conversant on such issues as a procedure's pain, side effects and recuperation, especially if the procedure is routinely prescribed. It would also be helpful if a pamphlet about the procedure were available.

Pain

It is ironic that as I am sitting here writing this section on pain, I am experiencing my topic firsthand. This round of pain began about two weeks ago, and it is surprisingly similar to the original problem that brought me to Dr. Meyer in the first place. Searing pain radiating down both sides of my back to my lower back and across the front in the breast area. Rather than striking intermittently throughout the day, the pain is constant, sometimes bringing me to tears. In addition, the one thing that is different this time is that it is in my stomach as well, making it hard to eat, drink or even sit in a comfortable position.

When I told Dr. Miller about it, he ordered a nerve block to be done. This is where a surgeon—with a l-o-n-g thin needle—goes into the *celiac axis* (a group of nerves that lies between the pancreas and the spine) and injects alcohol into the nerves to deaden them. Just like with the biopsy, I wanted to be put to sleep for the procedure, but I had to be awake enough to tell the surgeon what I was feeling inside, so I agreed to twilight sleep. This time, everything from the duration of the procedure to the agreeableness of the doctor and nurses went well. The only thing that failed was the block itself! It didn't provide me with adequate relief, and I went back on painkillers. Some people can have more than one nerve block, but, in my case, it was decided that I would not have another one because my dying body was too frail. I almost cried when I heard the news, but then I decided that becoming resigned to painkillers took less energy than being angry at my frailty.

Being in pain is one of the cancer patient's greatest fears, and it is a fear that is well justified. Whether the pain is radiating, pulsing, burning or feels like sharp stabbing jolts, it affects every part of the person's life, not just the physical body. Quality of life for the cancer patient becomes based upon freedom from pain.

The Issue of Prognostication ...

... Or should I say "time"? The reality of dying, ultimately your death, boils down to running out of time. Few issues in the end-of-life field are more crucial and controversial than offering a terminally ill patient the timeline to his death.

Our society emphasizes making the most of each second on a 24/7 basis. Society frequently judges a person by how much has been accomplished within a given period of time. But to a dying person, time takes on a more encompassing feeling because the end of time—death—is when a person is measured for life accomplishments, not just individual conquests.

When a terminally ill diagnosis is handed down to a patient, everything in that person's world is measured in days, hours, minutes and seconds. Because the threat of death is so traumatic, the dying person will bring everything into the present without thinking of the future. That's why the answer to "How long do I have?" is so crucial to the dying patient. The answer clarifies and gives a foundation upon which to complete life's final tasks.

But the controversy in prognostication lies in the inability of doctors to accurately present the future to the dying patient. As Nicholas Christakis and Elizabeth Lamont of the University of Chicago Medical Center found out in their 2000 study on prognostication, only 20 percent of predictions for 468 patients were accurate. The majority (63 percent) was overoptimistic, with 17 percent being overpessimistic. Those who gave the most optimistic predictions were doctors who had known their patients for a long time and established a relationship with those persons.[11]

• • • • • • • • • • • • • • • • • • •

While there are some diseases, such as heart disease and chronic obstructive pulmonary disease, where accurate prognostication is difficult, some illnesses like cancer have very predictable and established timelines. What hampers the doctors' abilities to accurately plot the course of an illness is the absence of training and published literature to help them formulate their predictions. Ironically, while prognostication is probably one of the most important components in end-of-life care for the dying person, the medical field tries to ignore or cover it up.

Prognostic errors can have serious effects on the quality of care given to dying patients. Not only does producing overoptimistic predictions create false hopes for the patient,[12] but these predictions can prevent dying patients from getting the appropriate care. For example, one of the criteria for entering hospice is that the person is going to die within six months. An overoptimistic prognosis prevents the patient from accessing hospice care, which would enhance the quality of life until the end. As a result, dying patients receive only one month of hospice care rather than the ideal three months. In addition, inaccurate prognoses might lead the dying person to make choices that are counterproductive, such as seeking more treatment.

As a final note on prognostication, there is nothing more frustrating for this dying patient than to ask, "How long do I have?" and to hear my doctor say, "I don't know." Prognostication is a valuable component of end-of-life care. "Discussion of prognosis should remain an ongoing consideration during any treatment planning, including when there is evidence of advanced disease," write Joanne Lynn and Joan Harrold in their book, *Handbook for Mortals: Guidance for People Facing Serious Illness*.[13] In addition, there are several tools available to physicians that can guide them in making a prognostic decision. The single most important predictive factor is *functional ability*, a measure of how much patients can do for themselves. For example, the more time a patient spends in bed, the less favorable the survival time.[14]

Dying people have the right to know about the course of their disease. Because there is inadequate training for doctors in this ability, perhaps the answer lies in obtaining a second opinion on prognosis so this need of the dying patient would be satisfied.

· · · · · · · · · · · · · · · · · · · ·

Doctor/Patient Communications

Most health care professionals do not know how to talk to their patients about death and dying. Time and time again, with my hospice patients, family members and myself, I have seen doctors skirt the issue and divert any questions about dying to treatment issues. This leaves the patient confused and frustrated as well as gives false hopes.

"If there is nothing to discuss about death, then I'm not dying, right?" thinks the patient.

Just as true hope is crucial to a patient's well being, false hope can be destructive and malicious. By not telling a patient the truth about the illness— or worse yet, deliberately sugarcoating a diagnosis—a false relationship is created between the health care professional and the patient that is detrimental to both sides.

The Language of Dying

A person doesn't have to be newly-diagnosed to be confused by the language of medicine. Even long-term patients are befuddled by words such as *malignancy* and *carcinogenesis*, both of which mean the same thing: cancer. Many wonder, "What is the difference between discomfort and pain?"

"The language of dying was neither as clear nor as specific as it might usefully be," concluded the Institute of Medicine's 1997 report, "Approaching Death: Improving Care At The End of Life."[15] Because there is no universal wordage to describe an illness or its treatments, many patients and family members are frightened by the implications of other terminology.

When the language isn't clear, the patient becomes more confused and apprehensive in large part because the patient can't understand what the doctor is saying. This is particularly crucial in the initial stages of the disease when treatments, prognosis and general knowledge about the disease are tantamount.

It would serve both the doctors and the patients well if a common language were used when discussing medical cases. This way, everyone would "be on the same page" and hear the same thing, reducing the risk of confusion and misinterpretations at this critical stage for the patient. Some Internet sites, such as Breastcancer.org, have taken the first step towards this goal and have

• • • • • • • • • • • • • • • • • • •

developed a "Celebrity Talking Dictionary" to help anyone concerned about breast cancer hear, understand and use the key words related to this disease. Don't underestimate the power of building a universal language in the medical arena. Its influence touches every aspect of good medical care, from first diagnosis to doctor/patient communications.

For Doctors: Setting the Ground Rules of Doctor/Patient Communications

- Ask the patient, "How much do you want to know?"
- Give honest information on the disease, including prognosis. Emphasize that the prognosis may change during the course of treatment.
- Appoint someone on your staff to act as a contact person if the patient has any questions or concerns regarding nonmedical death-related issues.
- Send a card a month after you've given the diagnosis to show that you are there for the patient and family members.
- Schedule short check-in meetings with the patient. This can be done over the phone. Don't rush the conversation.
- Have a folder with printed materials handy to give to the patient. Included in this folder should be information that addresses key end-of-life concerns: hospice, *palliative care* (comfort care without trying to cure a terminally ill person), pain management, Medicare and personal finances, and advance directives. These documents can be easily obtained from a wide variety of organizations. Research the Web, your local library, your phone book and other sources for up-to-date information.

Working on the theory that four ears are better than two, many patients bring someone along to be their eyes and ears during crucial medical conversations; however, if the other person is emotionally involved, or particularly sensitive, this plan might not work to the benefit of the patient.

. . . .

Joe was with me when I received my diagnosis, and while I found his presence comforting and essential, I later learned that he heard the doctor in the same way that I did—about every other sentence. The same was true when my mother was diagnosed with congestive heart failure. Joe and I went together to meet with her doctor, and the whole time the doctor was talking, my mind kept thinking one sentence: "My mother is dying." It took a follow-up meeting complete with tape recorder for all three of us to get the facts straight.

Lessons Learned: Medical Issues

- Patients, who should be preparing for the end of life, might not be able to process the information fast enough to keep pace with events or might remain in denial.
- Each illness is unique in terms of characteristics, treatment, prognoses and survival rates. Comparing different kinds of cancers only serves to depress and isolate dying patients.
- The guidelines and standard practices that cover the healthy person should not be applied to the terminally ill. Dying people have their own special needs that are frequently ignored or bypassed because the rigid health care system "doesn't do it that way."
- Doctors often form a relationship with the disease and not the patient. Special attention should be paid to getting to know the patient in terms of behaviors and feelings rather than just identifying the patient as "the pancreatic cancer in Bed 5."
- Depression and anxiety are not the same thing. Medications aimed at treating anxiety, such as Ativan and Xanax, should be automatically considered as part of the initial treatment regimen.

• • • • • • • • • • • • • • • • • • •

8

Confusion and Transfusions

Perhaps what is most frightening than all of the horrors that chemotherapy and the doctors can do to a person is when your body turns against itself. That's what happened to me after the third round of chemo.

Dad, Joe and I were sitting downstairs, talking about Joe's morning golf game when suddenly, I felt "peculiar." My head began swimming, and I had no energy, not even to put my glass of water on the table. My first reaction was "I have to get to bed," so I abruptly stood up and headed for the stairs. I was able to take four steps before I collapsed. Joe was able to get me to sit on the toilet in our powder room until we figured out what to do. By this time, I had no control over my body. I was just one big gelatinous blob, but mentally I was very aware of what was going on. We were all terrified. Why was this happening? Is the pancreas secreting some hormone that is having this effect? Or is the problem the chemo?

I was so desperate to get to bed that Joe tried to get me up from the toilet slowly. I hugged him, as if we were doing a slow, sensual dance. The next thing I knew I was back on the toilet. I had totally passed out. This time, once I came to, we decided to wait a longer period of time until I felt stronger. Then, step by small step, we made our way to the staircase where Joe was able to get me up the stairs.

The first thing we did when I got into bed was take my vital signs. My blood pressure was 50/20 and my pulse was over 100. At least that explained a few of the reasons why I passed out. Realizing that I had made it safely to bed, Joe let his guard down. "I've been so scared for the past six weeks," he said, and we hugged and cried together for 20 minutes. It was one of the most intimate moments in our marriage.

When I told Dr. Miller about this episode, he said it was due to *dehydration*. A common problem in dying patients, dehydration occurs when a person doesn't take in enough fluids to maintain metabolic balance in the body. Blood pressure drops, nausea and lightheadedness are all symptoms of dehydration. I didn't realize how important dehydration was until this incident. After every chemo session, the nurses give me saline intravenously through my port, and I thought this was enough. What I didn't realize is how much chemo dries out the body, so intake of fluid is crucial. Afterward, I made a concerted effort to drink at least six glasses of fluid a day: water, juices, soups and ice pops. And I started to get out of bed very slowly for fear of collapsing again.

When I get closer to dying, my need for fluids will change, and I will need less hydration because my organs won't be able to handle tremendous amounts of fluids. Joe will have to give me small sips of fluids, ice chips or flavored mouth swabs instead.

There is a hidden side to illness, one that is rarely talked about. While people might talk about "side effects" loosely, the reality of what is involved is often hidden and circumspect. Learning there is a new side effect to treatment is equally upsetting and nerve wrecking. Each week, I have to have blood work done to be sure that my white and red blood cells are weathering the chemo adequately. All was going well until the day that Suzanne, the head nurse, came back with the most recent results.

"You need a blood transfusion *now*," she said. While a normal person's red-cell count is between 100,000 – 150,000, mine came in at 17,000, far too low for my blood to carry oxygen throughout my body. I wasn't too surprised to hear that something was wrong because I hadn't been feeling well. I was feeling extremely tired, and my legs felt like lead weights. It was getting harder and harder to climb the stairs at home, and all I wanted to do was sleep. Whenever I laid down, I fell into a deep sleep instead of watching TV or reading. I didn't call the doctor's office because I thought it was all part of the chemo routine. We hadn't been told of any unusual side effects to report, so we didn't know any better.

It was imperative that I get the transfusion ASAP to bring my body back to normal.

I'm finding this out as I'm going for my third transfusion in a month. Before my last chemo, I learned that my red-cell count was dangerously low. As a result, because the *red blood cells* carry oxygen throughout my body, it was becoming increasingly important to have two pints of A+ fused into my body.

. . . .

Having a blood transfusion for the first time is frightening. In addition to worrying about transmitted diseases (which, while precautions have minimized the risk, fear is still present because "nothing is perfect") there are all sorts of potential side effects related to the transfusion, such as shortness of breath, back pain, nausea and dizziness, to name a few. I couldn't help but think, "Don't I have enough to worry about" without being concerned about side effects from the transfusion?

So, Joe and I went to the hospital immediately to have my blood crossed and matched. Because it was late in the day, it was decided to do the transfusion first thing in the morning. This puzzled me because it appeared to be so urgent to have it done. But we got our answers the next day.

We arrived at 9 a.m. sharp, and we were led to a special room right off the Intensive Care Unit where the staff ratio is one-to-one. It took the nurse 30 minutes to explain all the complications and potential risks, including death, associated with a blood transfusion.

Despite my apprehension, the transfusion went well even though the six hours it took to do the job was long and tiring. The nurses monitored my vital signs every 15 minutes. I felt so much peppier afterwards. But this feeling of well-being didn't last long. One week later, my platelets started disappearing. Chemo was eating them up as well. *Platelets* are "the building blocks of blood," and their main function is to prevent bleeding by clotting. Without an adequate number of platelets in my system, I was told that I was at high risk of bleeding to death. I wasn't allowed to shave my legs, and I had to be careful around anything sharp. In addition, I was told to brush my teeth lightly (if at all) because bleeding in the gums is a common problem.

So, once again, Joe and I went back to "the girls" at Montgomery General Hospital to get the platelet transfusion. At this point in my treatment, my attitude was "I better die of the cancer I have suffered with, instead of something else."

Few patients realize there is a difference between transfusions. Physicians typically order the transfusion without explaining to the patient what is involved. Without good blood, chemo can't happen. To the dying person, this translates into being forced into new medical "territory" without having the knowledge to calm any fears or trepidation.

. . . .

9

Dying is a Team Effort

The irony of my situation has not passed me by. I'm the medical person in our family, the one who gives our dog allergy shots, who monitors blood pressure and who understands prescription directions. My husband, on the other hand, is the mechanical expert of the household. Give him a screwdriver or a drill, and he can do anything.

So the only way to approach his new role as my "nurse" was for us to frame his job differently. He was not my nurse—he was *my mechanic!* He learned to take "me" out of the picture and put total concentration on the catheter and pump used to infuse my chemo. By treating "me" like a piece of equipment, Joe is able to disconnect my catheter beautifully and in a very professional way. He carefully takes the tape off, unscrews the connection between the catheters, and then flushes the catheter out, first with saline, and then with heparin to keep the line open. Finally, he closes the clamp to the catheter and then goes downstairs for a small drink to calm his nerves.

Doing chemo at home is better than having it in the hospital, but it isn't without tremendous stress to both Joe and me. For Joe, it's the strain of "playing nurse," fearing that he is going to hurt me in some way. For me, being tethered to a pump at home makes it frustrating and difficult to go to the bathroom or climb stairs alone, but those are small annoyances. If I were in the hospital, all I would do is lie in bed, hooked up by a long IV apparatus that would allow me to go the portable toilet by the bed. What would be lacking is the loving and caring attention that I receive from my husband, my Dad, and even our dog, Gracie. One of my oncology nurses gave me valuable advice when she said, "It's amazing what a person can get used to when you have to," and that is certainly true for me and chemo at home. These annoyances are a small price to pay for not only getting more time at home, but also spending quality time with Joe. When he disconnects me, it is (in a weird way) a very intimate time for us. We are both scared and apprehensive, and we talk each other through the process.

• • • • • • • • • • • • • • • • • • •

The role of caregiver at a time like this is so important and vital, but it does come at a high price.

Sometimes I don't know which is worse—to be the dying person who is in God's hands or the caregiver who shares in every fear and torment, knowing that ultimately life will be without the loved one. I can't imagine being without Joe, and the separation that we are facing is overwhelming both of us.

Not that we have much of an equal partnership together now; all of the responsibilities of the house and my care are on his shoulders, and I worry about his health. His one outlet is golf, but he cancelled his game today because of my passing out. I'm trying to think of ways of minimizing his stress, but he is so protective of me.

Documenting my illness gives me an opportunity to really see myself as I am, and it is very upsetting. Hunched over, with my bald head hanging down, I do wonder if this is part of the meaning of suffering. I'm not contributing anything to anyone anymore. My care is a lot of work and I feel worthless and time consuming. If I had the energy to do just one thing to take the load off of Joe's shoulders, I would be happy.

From Joe: My Perspective

When Laura was diagnosed with pancreatic cancer, I knew that our lives had changed. Everything that used to be normal in our life no longer was. Our marriage was always based on teamwork. We both did household chores, shopping and cooking. As her disease progresses, the responsibility for these things is shifting more in my direction, and a new task has been added—taking care of her.

My definition of "caregiver" has its roots in my upbringing. I grew up in an area where the entire extended family—grandparents, aunts and uncles, siblings and cousins—all lived in the immediate area. When someone in the family was sick, the family provided whatever was needed. Meals were cooked and delivered, children were watched over and whatever the need was, it was taken care of. Because of this, my natural instinct is to "circle the wagons and close in the fences."

I had several caregiving experiences in my life before this. Although not in a hands-on way, I was involved when Laura's aunt in New York was dying from cancer. Laura's mother had moved in with her sister to take care of her, and Laura spent most weekdays in New York helping out. I would go to New York and help out during the weekends Laura didn't come home. I ran a lot of errands from grocery shopping to picking up prescriptions. I was an observer of the care Laura and her mother were providing.

I became more involved when Laura's mother was dying, and we brought her into our house to take care of her. During this period I played more of a direct role to help Laura and give her breaks. Many of the things I did were practical in nature such as cooking or changing the bed, but I was also able to do things to make Mom's life easier, like running her oxygen line through adjoining walls so she could move from the bedroom to the den without a problem.

Armed with this experience, I now found myself as Laura's primary caregiver. I was driven by my love for Laura. Knowing that I had to be strong for both of us, I was determined to give her the best possible care.

I was a caregiver on several levels. The first level was the easiest; handling the logistical issues of medical appointments, tests and treatment were just scheduling issues. The next level proved to be more complex.

I was uncomfortable with the concept of doing part of the chemotherapy at home. Patty, the home health care nurse assigned to do the hookup for the home infusion, had walked me through the procedure of disconnecting the pump and flushing the catheter. And she left detailed notes. Despite all this, I was concerned about what could go wrong. I had no doubt in my ability to follow directions, but it was unnerving nonetheless. The home infusion took eight hours and usually ended at midnight. If something went wrong, or if Laura had a reaction, I was going to have to rely on calling the phone number on the magnet on the refrigerator. Doing chemo at home was certainly more comfortable for Laura, so I put my reservations behind me.

The emotional level was the hardest to deal with. My wife was dying! It was my responsibility to make sure that her wish for a good death was fulfilled and to do whatever it took to make that happen. It was the most important undertaking I had faced in my life, and I was committed to doing it to the best of my abilities.

. . . .

My first thoughts were that I could handle everything by myself. "After all," I said, "Laura is my wife, and I am supposed to take care of her." Friends would ask if they could help, and my response would be that I had everything under control. This was a true statement in the beginning. In the first weeks following her diagnosis, the only change in our routine was a lot of doctor's appointments.

When I told my boss, Linda, about Laura's diagnosis, she immediately recommended that I speak with the human resources department. I was informed that I met the requirements of the Family Medical Leave Act. Because I was eligible, I was entitled to 12 weeks of leave to take care of Laura. An optional combination of paid and unpaid leave allowed me the flexibility to take off whenever I needed in order to take Laura to a medical appointment or take care of her at home. To make my life even easier, Linda also arranged for computer access for me so I could work from home.

As time went on, I realized that the role of caregiver was more complex than just taking care of Laura. It was requiring me to manage multiple tasks at the same time. I was taking care of her, trying to work, run errands, schedule medical appointments and monitor medications. Laura and I came up with a set of caregiver rules that soon helped to make my life a little easier. I just needed to open up and allow others to help.

Caregiver Considerations

The Caregiver Also Needs Care

In order to take care of a loved one, the caregiver needs to take care of himself or herself. Proper sleep and nutrition are essential elements. Time away from the patient is also important. There is nothing wrong with taking a break and doing something for your own relaxation, providing there is someone to stay with the patient. There is no reason to feel guilty about having dinner out with friends, seeing a movie or playing a round of golf. Activities will give the caregiver a physical and mental break from the stress of the situation.

I took advantage of having Dad in the house to spend some time out of the house, usually to play an occasional round of golf with friends or to go to a Washington Redskins football game. I also relied on friends to get some down time. Even if I didn't leave the house, having someone with Laura gave me the chance to relax.

． ． ． ． ． ． ． ． ． ． ． ． ． ． ． ． ． ． ．

Taking breaks helps avoid any resentment on the part of the caregiver. Although the patient is the one dying, the caregiver is also suffering in her or his own way. The impending loss of a loved one is a devastating position to be in, and it is not always easy to keep things in a proper perspective.

Taking breaks can also provide a meaningful opportunity for the patient. When Laura was capable, she would go out to lunch with friends, or we would arrange for a friend to take her to a routine medical appointment, and afterwards, they would go out for lunch. It allowed her to maintain a bit of a normal life, while giving me some time for myself.

It is worthwhile to take advantage of available resources. In our case, Laura's oncologist had a therapist on staff that was available to meet with us together and individually. Many hospice groups have counselors on staff to assist the caregiver and family members. Clergy members are another valuable resource.

Open up to others and use available resources.

I was reluctant at first to take people up on their offers to help. Having someone pick up groceries, run errands or bring over a prepared meal allowed me to spend more quality time with Laura. It also gave me the opportunity to use the time to relax. As time went on, I realized how much help this was to me. (Looking back at the schedule I was keeping, I'm not sure how I did it.)

In the beginning when Dad was staying with us, I would leave the house and go to work around 6 a.m. If Laura had a doctor's appointment, I would leave work, go home to take her to the appointment, take her back home, and go back to work. On the chemo days, I would go to work, then pick her up and take her to chemo, go back to work, then go back to pick her up and go back home. I eventually realized that the "back and forth" was too much. While I was not going to miss a chemo appointment, transfusion, major test or examination, I began to let close friends, primarily Julia, take Laura to routine blood tests. This "team approach" took a lot of pressure off me.

Adapt to change. Things that used to be priorities aren't that important.

As our lives had changed when Laura was diagnosed, everything else also changed. In the grand scheme of things, it really didn't make any difference if things weren't perfect. We learned to not worry if the house wasn't cleaned and vacuumed before company came over. It didn't make a difference if the lawn was mowed on time. Priorities that used to be so important before the diagnosis were significantly diminished or simply ceased to exist.

It is okay to have a meltdown.

Laura and I never hid the fact that she was going to die. We both knew it, and although we didn't dwell on it, we tried to make sure that it didn't consume our lives. There were times when something would trigger a "reality moment," and I would break down. Although I tried to have these moments in private it wasn't always possible. Often times the meltdown would serve multiple purposes—the emotional release was good for me, and it usually led to a good conversation between us.

Do not feel stupid if you have to ask a lot of questions.

Meeting with doctors can be an overwhelming experience. The best advice we were given at the onset was either to take a tape recorder to doctors' appointments, or bring someone else along with us. Laura and I learned very quickly that even though we were in the same place at the same time, we heard different things. Neither of us could ever recall all that was said during a consultation without listening to the tapes or reading notes that we or someone else had taken. We followed up on any points that weren't clear.

Asking questions is extremely crucial when dealing with treatment. Although we were given a lot of information about the side effects of chemotherapy, there were always things that cropped up that we weren't expecting. We never assumed that a reaction was "normal." If we had any questions or concerns, we immediately called the doctor. We also would check with other resources to get as much information and insight as possible merely to complement what we learned.

Several times we called our general practitioner, Dr. Meyer, to ask his opinion on something or to get a clarification on something we were told. The best example of this occurred when Dr. Kaplan, Laura's second oncologist, called on a Friday evening to give me the preliminary test results showing that the cancer had spread into Laura's back and possibly her brain. He also wanted to do another follow-up test to confirm the cancer's presence in more locations. I asked him if he thought I should tell her, and his response was to wait until after the final test was done the following Wednesday and we had confirmation.

I could understand why he felt that way, and at first I also thought that it was the prudent thing to do. Laura was sleeping at the time, and I sat there trying to process the information. I realized two things. First, Laura would want to know this. Second, I knew that it would be tough for me to keep this information to myself for the next several days. I called Dr. Meyer to ask his opinion. I tearfully recounted my conversation with Dr. Kaplan, and without hesitation he told me I had to tell Laura. He said that it would be unfair for me to carry this knowledge alone, but more important, Laura would kill me if she found out that I knew and didn't tell her.

I learned very quickly that it is important to ask questions of the hospice provider. I learned to question everything from the timing and dosage of medications to whether it was okay to leave expired pain patches on Laura because removing them was painful.

Our health insurance provider had assigned a case manager to monitor Laura's treatment and assist with any issues that arose. Speaking with her, I was able to get the home health care aide to come to the house five days a week rather than the three days that hospice recommended.

Choose One Doctor to be a Main Point of Contact
We were dealing with a variety of doctors during Laura's illness—oncologists, radiologists and specialists. We were receiving information and recommendations from all of them. We found it best to use one doctor, in our case Dr. Meyer, to filter the information for clarification. Choose the doctor with whom you have the best relationship and who is willing to help.

. . . .

10

Calm Before the Storm

The period from mid-fall through the holidays was transitional for Laura and me. PET-scan results showed that her tumor was shrinking, but the chemotherapy was taking a massive toll on Laura. It was taking her longer to recover from each round of chemo, and it had gotten to the point that by the time she started regaining her strength, it was time for another round. Each round of chemo was depleting her red blood cells, and as a result she was undergoing whole blood transfusions and platelet transfusions.

We met with Dr. Miller, Laura's first oncologist, in October to discuss Laura's treatment. Laura and I had already decided that quality of life was the most important issue for us. The longer recovery period was not giving Laura enough time to write, and it was giving us very little time to do anything for ourselves. We were planning to ask Dr. Miller if the treatments could be moved to every third week. This would give us an additional week where Laura would be stronger and allow us more time to do things.

Dr. Miller told us what we already knew. The treatment was shrinking the tumor, but Laura was paying a high price. To our surprise, he recommended that the treatments be spaced four weeks apart. We asked him what impact that would have on how much time Laura would have, and he said he was unable to tell. We all agreed that given the option we would choose quality of time rather than length of time.

In mid-October, Dad went back to Florida. He needed to get back to his life for a while, and Laura and I were glad to have the time alone. Although Dad was a big help to us, having someone in the house 24 hours a day was tough. It gave us little privacy. There were times that Laura and I would want to talk privately, and we felt bad leaving the room. We weren't trying to exclude Dad from conversation, but there were times we just needed to talk about things we weren't willing to share at that moment. Because it had been several weeks since her last treatment, Laura had begun to regain her strength.

• • • • • • • • • • • • • • • • • • • •

We decided to take advantage of this and go away for a few days. We were limited in where we could go because sitting in the car for long periods of time was uncomfortable for Laura. We decided that we would go back to the Homestead.

Laura's Homestead Memories

It was on our "honeymoon" 15 years ago that I introduced Joe to our special escape haven, the Homestead Resort. I put honeymoon in quotes because it wasn't the traditional escape that most newlyweds experience. Because we were married on December 23, 1988—two days before Christmas—our postceremony plans had to include both sides of our new united family. A large part of why Joe and I were married was because of our love of family, and this commitment made it a special holiday.

So, we spent Christmas Eve with Joe's family at his brother John's house in Reading, Pennsylvania. It gave me a golden opportunity to better know my new father- and mother-in-law, as well as John's family (wife Mary Ellen, son Jamie and daughter Lisa). The next day, Joe and I left to spend Christmas with my mother and brother, Willy, who were already at the Homestead.

Located in the mountains of Virginia near the West Virginia line, the Homestead has played a large role in my life. Both my grandmother and mother had stayed there many times, and my aunt and uncle would spend a week each year being spoiled by the resort's amenities. This Christmas, I was checking in with my new husband!

Throughout our marriage, whenever things got tense or too stressful, Joe and I would go to the Homestead, gradually making it our "home away from home." As a result, we have gotten to know many of the staff. The Maitre d', Woody Pettus, has been at the Homestead for 48 years and every time I see him, I think of my grandmother being seated by him. And we remember Felicia, Woody's heir, on her first day on the job in the early 1990s. The third person in our inner triumvirate, Oswald, is the waiter who never smiles. One of the most efficient and courteous waiters, Oswald is known for not smiling.

So, with these three to look forward to, it was only natural that when I received my devastating diagnosis, Joe and I would turn to the Homestead for comfort and solace. And regrouping.

* *

Joe's Thoughts

The long weekend was just what we needed. As was usually the case, we would have breakfast on the balcony, read the newspaper, and decide what we would do that day. We spent time at the pool, took walks through the gardens and browsed the shops in town, where we did some Christmas shopping. Although it wasn't a conscious decision, we really didn't talk about Laura's illness. We talked instead about what we were going to do for the upcoming holidays.

We told Woody and Felicia about Laura's illness, and they went out of their way to accommodate us. In the dining room the first night, Laura didn't eat much of her dinner, and Oswald asked her if the food was satisfactory. Laura replied that everything was fine, but that she didn't have much of an appetite.

The next evening, Laura looked at the menu, and the only items she showed an interest in were appetizers. Two of her favorites were being served—smoked salmon and Alaskan crab claws. None of the entrées appealed to her, so she asked Oswald if she could just have the two appetizers. Never smiling, he said he would take care of her and brought her the crab claws as an appetizer and the salmon as an entrée.

Oswald greeted us for breakfast the next morning and escorted us to our table. He asked how our evening was and how Laura was feeling. He then broke into a wide grin and said to her, "If nothing on the breakfast menu appeals to you, I'm sure I can find smoked salmon or anything else you might want in the kitchen." As we left, he gave Laura a big hug.

Leaving to return home was a bittersweet moment. Although neither one of us said it aloud, we both wondered if we would ever return. Going home meant going back to reality. It was back to blood tests and chemotherapy, but it also meant planning for Thanksgiving and Christmas. Dad would be coming back a few days before Thanksgiving and staying until after the New Year.

When we returned home Laura told me that she wanted to preplan her funeral. Her reason for doing this was based in part on her experience when her aunt died in New York. The morning after her aunt died, Laura had to meet with the funeral director to make arrangements. Although Laura knew what her aunt's wishes were, it was a difficult and emotional ordeal to pick out a casket, arrange for the service and choose appropriate prayer cards. Based upon this experience, Laura opted to make prearrangements for her mother's funeral.

Now Laura was doing her best to protect me from going through this ordeal after she passed away. The representative from the funeral home came to our house, and we went through the whole process with Laura describing what kind of service she wanted and picking out the urn that would hold her ashes. Laura and I had decided that we wanted to be interred in a double urn, and it was comforting for both of us to know that someday we would both be together again. It was a surreal moment when Laura signed the consent form for her own cremation.

By doing this before the need was real, our efforts became a less emotional event and more of a business transaction.

Nightline

Laura and I got involved with *Nightline* in the autumn of 2003. Producers were originally doing a story on Terri Schiavo, the woman in Florida who was the center of a conflict between her husband and her family. She had severe brain damage and did not have a living will or advance directive. Ms. Schiavo's family was arguing over what her wishes were, with one side saying she did not want to be kept alive by artificial means and the other side saying the opposite. This conflict was exactly why Laura was an advocate for patients' rights and highlighted the need for people to make their wishes known to their loved ones. *Nightline* producers had called Dr. Joanne Lynn, an expert in end-of-life issues and a good friend of Laura's, to solicit people to speak on this subject. Joanne explained Laura's situation and suggested they contact her.

The *Nightline* crew spent a lot of time with us in October and November. They conducted interviews at our house and chronicled Laura's chemotherapy and tests. The crew was attuned to Laura's illness and made certain that they were not overly intrusive. The original program aired in early December, and we watched it with nervous anticipation.

Just before the program aired, Laura said to me "What if it's not good?" We agreed that based on the compassion of the *Nightline* people involved, we were pretty certain that it would be a positive piece. And it was. Laura was very

• • • • • • • • • • • • • • • • • •

proud of her involvement in this project because she was adamant about getting across her message about having "a good death" and the importance of advanced directives and health care powers of attorney. This program got that message to a broad audience.

Laura's new chemo schedule was such that she would have almost two full weeks to recover before Thanksgiving. We decided to do what we usually did, which was host the holiday at home. We invited Brian and Kathy (our dear friends who introduced us) to come over with our seven-year-old godson, Sean, and his four-year-old sister, Aimee, plus Willy, Laura's brother, and Carolee, a friend of Laura's. Laura was concerned about me doing all the work and felt guilty about not being able to help as much as she would have like to, but she was reassured when Carolee agreed to come over early to help cook and set everything up.

Laura's Thoughts on Thanksgiving

Today is what could be my last Thanksgiving. It should be a joyful time for me but it is not. That's because everyone is too tense and mindful of the fact that I have cancer. On holidays, my father-in-law telephones everyone in the family and a lot of his friends, to send best wishes. Each time he talks to someone, he comes over to me, and says somberly, "So-and-so is praying for you." After the third phone call, I'm ready to hit him!

I don't need to be reminded of my condition, and I am trying so hard to make this a truly thankful day. But when it is constantly thrown in my face that people "are praying for you," it makes me angry. I guess I feel that if I can try and forget the whole situation for at least one day, they can too. Why can't they just say, "Happy Thanksgiving" and leave it at that?

Many people feel they have to acknowledge a person's illness all the time. I think it is partly their feeling of "I don't know what to say, so I'll harp on the disease." For dying people, there are times when we would like to get away from the situation, and try to act like normal, healthy people. Especially on a day such as Thanksgiving, which has been historically a happy occasion, reminders of the reality of my life are intrusive and upsetting.

This spills over into interpersonal relationships in my family. For Thanksgiving, we always invite close friends in addition to Dad and my brother, Willy.

Carolee is coming over early to help with the cooking. We also invited Brian, Kathy and their kids. But Brian called this morning and said he had a cold and wasn't feeling too well. This is a major issue for cancer patients who are on chemo because we don't have healthy immune systems due to the treatment. So, I can't be around anyone who is sick with a cold, flu or anything contagious. If I should contract the germs, I could end up in the hospital and possibly die. Telling someone like Brian that he can't come to our house is really hurting me because I love Brian, and I want to see him. But there are times when a cancer patient has to make hard decisions in terms of friendship and social connectedness. So, the final plans are that Kathy is bringing the kids, and Brian will stay home waiting for our care package of turkey. It is one more reminder of how sick I am that I can't see the people I want to.

Joe Remembers

With Thanksgiving behind us, Laura and I set our sights on December. We had a long talk about what we were going to do. Bobby and Pat, Laura's cousins from Vermont, wanted to come for Christmas, and their daughter Sara and her husband, Elliott, were going to fly in from Wyoming. Other than Willy, they were the only immediate family with which Laura had any contact. We were thrilled they would be coming. Although we never said it out loud, we both knew this was probably going to be Laura's last Christmas. We were both determined to make it a memorable one. Laura was scheduled for chemo the beginning of December, so she would be at her strongest for the holidays.

With careful timing and a lot of luck we were able to cram a lot of things into the month of December. It seemed like Laura had to go for blood tests almost every day. She found that if she were able to rest for part of the day, she had the energy to do things. She wanted to have a festive holiday, so we did things like we always did. She took great joy in decorating the Christmas tree. Robin, a friend and fellow hospice volunteer, had come over to help decorate the tree. She and Laura spent a lot of time talking about many of the heirloom ornaments Laura's grandmother had brought over from Germany. It was a wistful reminder of her youth as she held some of them and reminisced about her childhood Christmases.

. . . .

I had noticed that Dad was very quiet and didn't help decorate the tree. I asked him what was wrong, and he said, "I miss your mother." Mom had died two years earlier, and I understood what he said. I responded, "I miss her too, but Laura's probably not going to be here next year, and we need to focus on 'now,' not the past or the future."

Laura threw herself into the holidays with as much energy as she could muster. Although she could no longer drive, she insisted on going Christmas shopping, and we would make short concentrated trips to the mall when her energy level was up.

The first December celebration was our anniversary. I had planned for us to celebrate our anniversary early because of a dinner we were having on the actual date. Unknown to Laura, I had made reservations at one of our favorite restaurants, and to surprise her, I ordered a stretch limousine and driver to take us there. It was one of the high points of the holidays! The limo was fully decked out with disco lighting and a moon roof with pinpoint lights it in. We rode in it like two kids, laughing and singing along with the Christmas songs playing on the sound system.

In years past, Laura and I always hosted a Christmas party. When I raised the question to her about having one this year, she was less than enthusiastic. Her main objection was she would not be able to do much in preparation for it. I convinced her that if we had it catered, there would be less work for us to do, and she reluctantly agreed.

The week before the party brought more doctor appointments. Laura had been having a pain in her chest, and we went to see Dr. Miller about it. He recommended a bone scan to see what was going on. The scan showed there were some cancer cells in her breastbone. Dr. Miller referred us to a radiological oncologist for a consultation. We scheduled an appointment for December 26. Laura and I agreed that we would keep this information to ourselves. We didn't want to cause additional concern for our family and friends just before the holidays.

The Christmas party came off without a hitch. Many of our friends pitched in and helped pick up the food and get the house ready. Laura rested most of the day, and her energy level was pretty high. We had invited our closest friends, including Carolee, Brian, Kathy and the kids, John Driscoll, who was the best man at our wedding, Robin, and Julia, who had been indispensable over the last few months. Many of Laura's hospice friends were there as well. We also invited some of Laura's closest friends from graduate school, and her advisor, Dana Cable. All of them had been in constant contact during Laura's illness, and most of them would play important roles in the days and months to come.

There was a festive atmosphere in the house with the scent of a fresh-cut Christmas tree, cheerful holiday tunes playing throughout the house, and the laughter of little children. Conversations centered on the upcoming holidays and the recent airing of *Nightline*. Laura was comfortably settled in the living room talking with people, and I spent the evening getting to know some of the people from Laura's professional life.

Later, when everyone was gone, Laura and I sat in the family room. The only light was coming from the fireplace and the Christmas tree. We talked about the party and agreed that everyone seemed to have a good time. Laura told me that the best part of the party was it allowed her to escape the reality of her illness, and for those few hours she felt normal. Despite her initial reluctance to have the party, she was very happy we did. It was a welcome respite for both of us.

Our wedding anniversary was coming up on December 23, and we decided to make that a special occasion by hosting an anniversary dinner and inviting the people who had been there 15 years ago. It would be nice to celebrate with Dad, John Driscoll, his daughters, Elizabeth and Amanda, Brian and Kathy, and Bobby and Pat, Laura's cousins.

We kept up an intense pace through Christmas Eve and Christmas Day. Laura insisted on doing things as we always did, including going to Brian and Kathy's on Christmas morning to deliver presents to the children. Although she knew this was the last holiday she would spend with us, she refused to let her disease hold her back. She took naps each day to preserve her energy.

We met with Dr. Ampe, the radiological oncologist, the day after Christmas. After reviewing the scans, Dr. Ampe recommended that Laura undergo radiation therapy. He was confident that it would alleviate a lot of the pain. Laura underwent the pretreatment measurements and scans, and we agreed that treatment would start the following Monday. The treatments went well. Laura suffered minimal side effects, and the radiation did help to reduce the pain.

• •

In early January, Laura began having a lot of pain in her back, and as a result, the doctor prescribed painkillers. Although they helped, the medications did not fully alleviate the pain, and they made Laura feel unsteady and spacey. Dr. Miller recommended that Laura have a nerve block done that she mentioned earlier. He recommended a doctor who had done the procedure many times. Laura and I then met with Dr. Meyer to discuss this procedure, and he recommended the same doctor. Although there was no guarantee that it would be 100-percent effective—or even work at all, we decided it would be worth a try.

The procedure was scheduled for a Friday morning. On Wednesday, I delivered the CAT and PET scans that would be used by the doctor. While I was at the hospital, I ran into the doctor who had done the biopsy on Laura. He recognized me, probably because he had seen the *Nightline* program, and asked how Laura was doing. I told him about the upcoming nerve block and went home.

When I arrived home, Laura told me the nerve block had been rescheduled from Friday to the following Monday because of a scheduling conflict. I immediately called the hospital to find out what was going on. After talking to several different people, I was told that the doctor I had spoken with at the hospital made the change so that he could do the procedure himself. I was livid!

I asked on whose authority the decision was made and I was told that when a doctor says to do something, it is not questioned. After several discussions with various people, I was told that the decision was made in order to provide "continuity of care for the patient." The assumption was made that because this doctor had done the biopsy, we would be more comfortable with him rather than a doctor we didn't know.

I stated that I had several issues with this. First of all, Laura had requested a specific doctor based upon the recommendation of her doctors. Secondly, because this procedure was to alleviate pain, delaying it by several days would result in her being in pain longer than necessary, and finally, didn't it make sense to discuss this with the patient rather than make a unilateral decision.

As Laura had feared, *decisions were being made for the patient without any input from the patient.* After several conversations, the procedure was rescheduled with the doctor we had originally requested.

* * * * * * * * * * * * * * * * * * * *

The nerve block was unsuccessful so Laura was back to taking painkillers. We met with Dr. Kaplan to discuss other options. (Dr. Kaplan had replaced Dr. Miller as Laura's primary oncologist because Dr. Miller went on an extended sabbatical.) Dr. Kaplan decided that the best course of action was to hospitalize Laura for several days to try and get her pain under control, and have more tests done to try and determine the cause of the pain. On February 1, Laura went back into the hospital and underwent another battery of CAT scans and MRIs.

Working with Physicians

Dealing with doctors can be a trying experience. Patients, caregivers and family members tend to put high demands on doctors. It is important to develop a relationship with the doctors that will achieve the desired results without alienating the doctor from the patient and family, or the family and the patient from the doctors. A time might arise when decisive action is required, and when that occurs, it is best to handle the matter in a way that will not upset the patient.

♦ ♦

11

Final Days

Dr. Kaplan called on Thursday, February 12, 2004, with results of the most recent MRI. It showed the cancer had spread to three areas in Laura's back, and it also confirmed that the cancer had spread to an area outside her brain. He suggested that we make an appointment with Dr. Ampe to discuss the possibility of undergoing radiation on her back to relieve the pain. I asked him what effect this new information had on her prognosis, and Dr. Kaplan said she probably had "a month or two." Laura and I discussed it and decided we would call Dr. Ampe in the morning. If radiation would reduce the pain in her back, we felt it would be worth trying.

I called Dr. Ampe's office on Friday morning and spoke with the nurse. She said she would get the most recent MRI films and give them to Dr. Ampe and call us after he had reviewed them. Less than an hour later, Veronica called back and asked how soon we could make it in. We agreed to be there by 11 a.m.

I helped Laura get out of bed and get ready to leave. Because of the pain and the medication, she was becoming unsteady. When we arrived, we were immediately taken to an examination room. After a consultation with one of the interns, Dr. Ampe came in. He explained that there was significant deterioration in the T12, L2 and L4 sections of Laura's spine, which was causing the pain. He recommended doing the radiation workup and calculations, and starting therapy immediately. A 10-day course of treatment would be required, and Laura would notice a decrease in pain after four or five treatments.

It took the better part of the day for the preparatory work to be done, and Laura was uncomfortable sitting and waiting. To help with her pain, they gave her Actiq, which is a fast-acting fentanyl lollipop that releases pain medication by sucking on it. The lollipop worked well, and they gave us a prescription for more.

· · · · · · · · · · · · · · · · · · · ·

While Laura was going through some preliminary measurements and a mock-up for the CAT scan, I went out to get us lunch. On the way to the hospital cafeteria, I ran into Dr. Kaplan. I told him that Laura was going to begin radiation. He told me that after Laura was through with her treatment she should go back to him to have blood work done and to plan for future chemotherapy. I had a feeling that we would not be seeing Dr. Kaplan again.

Laura finally had her first radiation treatment at 4 p.m. Friday. We were to return on Saturday afternoon for treatment, and with Sunday off, and resume daily treatments on Monday. Laura and I were exhausted when we finally left, and she fell asleep in the car on the way home.

The President's Day weekend was going to be busy for us. Willy was spending the night, and he and I were going out Saturday morning to buy bedroom furniture for his new assisted living apartment. Sara and Elliott were arriving Saturday afternoon from Wyoming to spend the weekend with us.

Robin and Willy were at the house when we got home. Laura was exhausted and really wanted to rest, but settled into her recliner to talk to Willy. Although we had been keeping Willy updated on Laura's condition, she was very protective of him and put up a brave front. We ordered a pizza for dinner, and shortly thereafter, Laura went up to bed. Willy had never seen the *Nightline* episode, so he and I watched it. When it ended, I tried to draw him into a conversation about it, but he didn't want to discuss it. He simply said it was "nice" and went to bed.

We had arranged for Robin to stay with Laura on Saturday morning while I took Willy furniture shopping. I had to be back home by 11 a.m. to take Laura to radiation, so Willy and I took off bright and early to go shopping. We arrived at the store and were immediately met by a salesman who offered to help us. I told him this was going to be the easiest sale he ever made and told him what we needed. Forty-five minutes later the sale was completed, Willy was on his way home via Washington's Metrorail subway, and I was headed back to the house.

The flowers I had ordered for Valentine's Day arrived while I was out with Willy. Although Laura loved them, she was upset because she wasn't able to get out and get me anything. I told her that having her here was the best present I could have.

· · · · · · · · · · · · · · · · · · · ·

Robin had helped Laura get up and dressed, and they were sitting in the family room talking when I got home. Laura looked tired, and she had very little energy. We left for radiation and arrived right on time. Because this was a Saturday, the office was technically closed; however, Chris, the technician who would do the treatment, had arranged to be there. He met us at the door and brought a wheelchair for Laura.

Dr. Ampe came into the office while Laura was getting ready for treatment. He told me to come into his office and began to show me images of Laura's spine on his computer screen. He told me that he was surprised at how much her condition had deteriorated since she was last there in early January. He explained that the cancer was eating away in areas of her spine, and as a result discs were compressing and threatening to collapse. This is what was causing the pain. I asked him if this was typical, and his response was that pancreatic cancer patients don't normally make it long enough for this to occur.

I then asked him if he was going to do anything about the area in her head. He told me that she would be gone before that became an issue. I told him that Dr. Kaplan's prognosis was a month or two, and he shook his head "no." I asked him, "We're looking at a couple of weeks, aren't we?" He replied, "Yes." My heart sank as I left his office to help Laura get dressed—but I appreciated his honesty.

Laura was exhausted when we got home, and I helped her get into bed to rest. Later that afternoon, Laura's cousin, Sara, and her husband, Elliott, arrived. It was great to see them, and I felt relieved having company in the house. I filled them in on recent events, and told them that Laura had changed considerably since they last saw her at Christmas.

Laura was awake when they went up, and she was truly happy to see them. Sara sat on the bed, and they chatted until Laura wanted to rest before dinner. Laura had been Sara's mentor and role model since Sara was little. Laura was determined to come downstairs and join us for dinner—and she did.

After dinner Laura went back to bed, and she and Sara talked more. There was always a strong bond between the two of them, and Laura enjoyed her company. When Sara came downstairs, she, Elliott and I talked about everything. They were both amazed at the change in Laura in the past two months, and they both realized this would probably be the last time they saw her.

· · · · · · · · · · · · · · · · · · ·

Time to Make Treatment Decisions

I was up early on Sunday morning. It was the one time of the day when the house was quiet. It was my time to relax, read the paper and collect my thoughts before things got busy. I thought about how weak Laura had become in the last few days and realized that continuing radiation was going to drain her energy even more. I thought about everything that Dr. Ampe had told me. It was becoming obvious that the time to make a decision regarding future treatments had come.

Laura awoke around 9 a.m., and I helped her downstairs. She settled into her recliner and said to me, "We need to talk." Laura knew she was past the point of any curative treatment, she said her primary concern was managing her pain. I asked her about going to radiation on Monday, and she responded that she wasn't sure she would be physically able to make it. I filled her in on my conversation with Dr. Ampe, and it was no surprise to me that she knew the cancer was out of control.

We both knew we had reached another turn in the path, but this time we knew exactly where the path was leading. I turned to her with tears in my eyes and said, "Sweetie, this is one of the hardest things I've ever had to say, but do you think it's time to stop treatment and concentrate on pain management?" We both began crying and hugged each other. When I was able to speak, I asked her if she wanted me to make arrangements to bring in hospice. She nodded "yes."

Laura and I sat and talked for a while longer. She wanted Dr. Meyer to take over her care at this point. She felt comfortable with him and was confident that he would do whatever he could to manage her pain. I helped her back upstairs to rest.

I called Dr. Meyer on his cell phone and filled him in on everything that had been going on. As always, he said he would take care of things and his staff would make the necessary arrangements and call me on Monday.

The rest of Sunday passed uneventfully. Sara and Laura spent a lot of time talking, and I took advantage of the opportunity to relax.

Monday was going to be a busy day. Dr. Meyer's office called to tell us that Community Hospice would come to the house on Tuesday to complete the intake process. I was disappointed at the news because I wanted hospice to

. . . .

come that day. I decided to call Dr. Joanne Lynn to see if she could expedite things. A while later, I got a phone call saying the hospice nurse would be out later in the afternoon.

Sara spent time trying to get Laura to eat and drink a little. Laura did not really eat on Sunday, but was occasionally taking sips of water or juice. Sara also washed Laura's face and made sure she was comfortable. Laura did not get out of bed Monday, except to go to the bathroom. Although she was tired, Laura was mentally alert and talkative. She perked up a lot when Dan Green from *Nightline* came to visit. He only spent a few minutes with Laura, but she and I were very grateful for his visit.

It was a very tearful goodbye when Sara and Elliott left Monday afternoon. Sara realized this would be the last time she saw Laura, and it was a painful parting for both of them.

The hospice intake nurse arrived around 4 p.m., and we spent the better part of the next hour going through the forms and introduction to hospice. She told me the regular nurse would come on Monday, Wednesday and Friday. She was also going to arrange for a health care aide to come to assist with bathing Laura.

I took the nurse upstairs to examine Laura, who was awake and able to talk with the nurse and answer questions for a few minutes. Afterwards, I asked the nurse how Laura was doing, and if she had any thoughts about how long Laura would linger. She said that it was hard to tell because this was the first visit. She said Laura's blood pressure was good, and her heart was strong. She discussed getting oxygen equipment to help Laura breathe and an alternating-pressure pad to help prevent bedsores. She recommended getting a hospital bed because it would be better for the pressure pad, and it would be more comfortable for Laura. I told her that Laura's wish was to die in her own bed, and I declined the hospital bed. She assured me that she would place the necessary orders.

I felt relieved knowing that hospice was involved. It was a comfort to know the nurse would be coming to the house every other day, and I would have help bathing Laura and getting her into fresh pajamas. It was also a relief to know there was someone a phone call away at any time of day.

◆ ◆ ◆ ◆ ◆ ◆ ◆ ◆ ◆ ◆ ◆ ◆ ◆ ◆ ◆ ◆ ◆ ◆

About Hospice Care

A hospice is an organization created to care for dying individuals in the last six months of life. There comes a time for many terminally ill patients when they will not benefit from nor will they be able to withstand any more curative treatment (trying to fight the disease). A decision must be made at this juncture as to where the patient will spend the remaining months or days. Hospitalization might not be an option if there is no treatment planned other than for pain management. The remaining options are putting the patient in a nursing home or staying at home. This is often a difficult decision to make, and it is dependent upon the patient's wishes and the family's willingness and ability to care for a loved one at home.

In our case, Laura had made it well known that she wanted to die at home, and I was determined to make that a reality. If the situation were reversed, I would have wanted the same thing.

The decision to call in hospice to assist at the end of life can be an emotional one for both the patient and the family. For many, it is at this point that they are forced to acknowledge and accept the fact that their loved one is going to die. This might also be true for the dying person. During the course of Laura's illness I always knew this day would come, and when it did I had to reluctantly accept the reality that we were entering the final phase of Laura's life. It is important to note that accepting this did not mean I was giving up. If anything, the hardest work for me was yet to come.

Hospices provide invaluable help to the patients and their families, but it is important to note that hospices *do not* take control from the patient and the caregiver.

The decision to put a loved one into hospice care is one that should be made between the patient, the family and the family doctor. Hospices are not necessarily all alike. Several hospices might serve the same geographical area. Some hospices are nonprofit while others are for-profit. Hospices might be affiliated with hospitals or religious groups. An inpatient facility at a hospital also might be available. In selecting a hospice, you should take the time to look into all of them to see which one is best for your needs. There are resources in the appendix of this book to assist you in obtaining information about hospice care and to help you locate resources in your area.

. . . .

Medical hospices do a tremendous job assisting patients and their families. Their primary goals are managing pain and keeping the patient comfortable. There are three requirements for admission into a medical hospice. The primary requirements are the patient has less than six months to live and is referred to hospice by a physician. The third requirement is no further curative treatment is planned.

Upon admission into hospice, an intake coordinator, usually a nurse, will visit the patient at home and do an assessment. This includes determining what medical equipment, such as hospital bed or oxygen equipment, the patient might need. Hospice will assist in having this equipment delivered to the home. Hospice will also coordinate with the patient's physicians to get the required medications. In many cases, hospice can also arrange for the medication to be delivered to the patient's home. The intake coordinator will also set up a schedule for regular visits by a hospice nurse. Many hospices also provide home health aides to assist with bathing and hygiene tasks.

Hospices have professionals on staff to assist both the patient and the caregiver. The professionals include social workers, pastoral professionals and counselors. They assist in many ways, from sending home health aides to talking with family members. In addition, hospices might follow up with the family after the patient dies and offer bereavement support in groups or personal contact.

Community hospices are not medical. They can provide volunteers who will assist the patient and family by visiting with the patient, running errands, and driving the patient to medical appointments. They also offer support to family members and provide bereavement counseling. Unlike medical hospices, nonmedical hospices do not require a physician's referral. Laura began her career in hospice with Hospice Caring, Inc., a non-profit, volunteer hospice.

Tuesday

When I awoke on Tuesday, Laura was still sleeping. I had given her pills at 4 a.m., and she had been sleeping peacefully since. I went up at 8 a.m. to check on her and give her medication. She had no energy and was not speaking. I called into work and informed Beth, my boss's assistant, of everything that had been going on, and that it looked like it would only be a couple of days. I told her I would not be going into work, but would keep her informed of what was going on.

Several people came by to visit Tuesday. Laura would open her eyes, but she said very little. Visitors would sit by the side of the bed and talk to her, but there was little or no response. One of the visitors was Denise Watterson, a friend of ours, and a professional acquaintance from Hospice of Frederick County here in Maryland. She spent a few minutes with Laura and came downstairs. We sat and talked for a while. I was having a tough time holding myself together, but I was trying to put up a brave front. Denise thought it probably wouldn't be too much longer.

I was beginning to think this was going to be the day I was going to lose Laura. Although I knew this moment would eventually arrive, I felt totally unprepared for it. It was hard to believe that she really was going to die. Early Tuesday afternoon, I called Kathy Diestch, a friend of ours who was the volunteer coordinator at Hospice Caring, and asked her to call a priest to come to the house and give Laura last rites.

Kathy and Nancy Ochsenreiter, another hospice friend, arrived, and we waited for the priest. They both stayed in the room while the priest prayed and gave Laura the sacrament. I sat at the bedside and held her hand. She awoke while the priest was there and seemed to understand what was occurring. When he was through, Kathy and Nancy walked the priest downstairs. I was too upset to leave the room, and I sat there crying and holding Laura's hand.

Dr. Meyer stopped by later Tuesday afternoon just to check on Laura. It had been years since I had heard of a doctor making a house call. It was comforting having him stop by. We talked for a few minutes after he saw Laura. He reminded me that if I needed anything, I could call him anytime.

The hospice nurse called late in the day. She would be making her first visit the next day, Wednesday. I filled her in on Laura's condition.

After Nancy and Kathy left, I called Pat Fry, Laura's cousin in Vermont. She had been a great source of information and advice, and I wanted to fill her in on everything that had been going on. I told Pat that I didn't think it would be much longer, and her advice to me was just relax and spend as much time with Laura as possible. I spent the rest of Tuesday lying on the bed next to Laura, holding her hand and watching television. When I went to sleep that night, I had no idea what the next day would bring.

· ·

Wednesday

Laura was awake and responsive on Wednesday. The night had been uneventful. As usual, she woke up around 4 a.m. and needed to go to the bathroom. Although she was weak, I was able to get her there and back into bed with no problem. After she took her pills, she went back to sleep.

We had a busy day ahead of us. The hospice nurse was due to arrive around 10 a.m. and the health care aide was due sometime before noon.

Janice, a friend from ABCD (Americans for Better Care of the Dying) and her teenage son, Conor, arrived to visit. She spent a little while with Laura, and then Conor went up. He had insisted that he had to come and see Laura. He spent a few minutes with her and then settled down in the family room with my electric guitar.

The hospice nurse, Sue, arrived around 10 a.m. She went straight up to Laura and gave her a short examination. Her blood pressure was good at 110/70, her pulse was strong, and her respiration was good. After the exam, I asked Sue if she knew when the pressure pad and oxygen would arrive. She called into the office and found out the order had never been placed. She assured me the order would be placed immediately. We talked about Laura's condition, and Sue told me that because this was her first visit, it was hard to make any judgments. Sue did say that she expected Laura to be in worse condition based upon what I had told her over the phone.

Shortly after Sue left, Helena, the health aide came. She was very gentle with Laura, giving her a sponge bath and changing her pajamas with minimal discomfort. Laura was exhausted from all the activity, and while I laid on the bed watching TV, she fell asleep.

The remainder of Wednesday was supposed to be quiet. Robin was going to stop by in the middle of the afternoon, and Carolee was going to stop by after work. They both understood that if Laura was sleeping, their visits would be short.

Laura was awake when Robin arrived. Robin sat by the bed, and they talked a little. I was downstairs when the phone rang. It was the medical-supply company asking if the oxygen and bed pad could be delivered right away. I said that would be okay, and went upstairs to tell Laura the equipment was coming.

* * * * * * * * * * * * * * * * * *

Laura was very interested in the delivery. She watched closely as the compressor, spare oxygen tanks and portable oxygen unit were brought in the room. As the deliveryman started to explain how to use the equipment, Laura broke in and said to me, "You pay close attention to him." She turned to Robin and told her to make sure I paid attention. She then asked the deliveryman his name. He responded, "Bob," and she said, "Bob, you make sure that he knows how to work this stuff." He promised he would.

For some reason, Laura was agitated, so Robin and I walked her to the den down the hall from the bedroom to sit down. I stayed with Bob and made sure I knew how to use the oxygen equipment. After he left, I took advantage of the situation and put the alternating-pressure pad on the bed and changed the sheets. When I went into the den, Laura and Robin were sitting and talking. Laura had calmed down, so I joined them for a while. A short while later, Laura went back to bed, and Robin left. Peace and quiet again—for a while.

Carolee came around 5:30 p.m. Wednesday afternoon and went up to see Laura. As was usually the case, I left the room and went downstairs so they could visit. After a few minutes, Carolee called me upstairs. Laura said that she wanted to talk to me alone, so Carolee went downstairs. I asked Laura if she wanted Carolee to leave, and she replied, "Yes." I went down and quickly filled in Carolee about our busy day, and she left.

I went back up to be with Laura, and she wanted to get up and get out of bed. I asked if she thought she could make it to the den again. I got her settled in the den and went to get her some ginger ale.

As we sat on the couch she said to me, "Do you want a divorce?" This took me aback, and it took me a few seconds to answer. I told her that was the furthest thing from my mind and asked why she would even think of such a thing. "There have been too many people in and out of here, and we're not spending enough time alone." I thought about what she said, and looking at all that had happened that day alone, I realized she was right. I promised her that we would cut down on the number of visitors and spend as much time alone as possible. While we were sitting there the phone rang several times. I looked at caller ID and told her who was calling, and her response each time was, "Let them leave a message." I was beginning to understand what she meant because in the span of about 30 minutes the phone rang four times.

* *

One of the calls was from John Driscoll. I knew why he was calling. He had been coming to the house a couple days a week to make dinner and was calling about that evening's arrangements. It was a great help to me because he would bring the food, cook and clean up. I wasn't allowed to do anything. I quickly took the call and told him not to come.

This extremely busy day made me realize I had another role to play. I had to become more aware of the number and timing of friends visiting Laura. Up to this point, if someone called and asked to visit, I had always asked Laura if it was okay. Now, it had become clear that too many visitors could be overwhelming for her, and I would have to limit the number of visitors and the duration of their stay.

This incident also highlighted difficulties in communication that sometimes occur. The patient's thought processes might be affected by the disease, the medications or both. In Laura's case, she would occasionally act out of character or say things that didn't make sense. These experiences are evidently normal, and it is important to remember that remarks or actions that seem unexpected or harsh should not be taken personally. As the patient has trouble communicating verbally, there are often other things that can communicate a powerful message. As it became harder for Laura to talk, a simple squeeze of my hand was her way of saying, "I love you."

As we were sitting in the den Laura said, "We have a room just like this at home." I said, "Sweetie, we are home—this is our den." She said it was like home, but it wasn't. I didn't know if the medication or the cancer made her say this. We stayed in the den a while longer, and I asked her if she was ready to go back to bed.

On the way back to the bedroom she saw the stairs and asked me, "Where do they go?" "Downstairs, to the kitchen and family room," I replied. She looked at me with an impish smile on her face and with the enthusiasm of a child going on an adventure said, "Let's go!" I wasn't about to argue with her, and although I was worried about getting her down the stairs and eventually back up, down we went.

I got her settled into her recliner and got her a small bowl of ice cream to eat. It had been a struggle to get her to eat anything the last few days, and I was happy to see her eat it. For the next hour or so, things were like the old days.

. . . .

We were sitting in the family room listening to music and talking. Even Gracie was happy. She had been going up to the bedroom several times a day and lying on the floor by the bed next to Laura. Now Gracie was lying on her bed next to her mom's recliner and happily accepting the treats Laura gave her. For me, it was the most relaxed I had been in days, and I enjoyed the moment.

We had been downstairs for about an hour when Laura said, "I want to call somebody." "Who do you want to call?" I asked. "Let's call Nancy." I dialed the number, and when Nancy Ochsenreiter answered, I simply said, "Somebody wants to talk to you," and handed the phone to Laura.

They had been talking for about 15 minutes when Laura asked me to get the calendar. She said to Nancy "Let's have lunch." She looked at the calendar and said, "I can't do it Thursday, how about tomorrow?" Before she hung up, I got on the phone with Nancy and confirmed that she was coming for lunch the next day. She told me she was totally taken by surprise by the phone call, and that when she left the house the previous day, she was convinced she would never see Laura again. Nancy subsequently said the phone call was a gift she never expected, and it had brought her incredible joy. Even in her final days, Laura had the ability to surprise and delight people.

Later, we called Bobby and Pat in Vermont, who were equally astonished. A little while after that, I helped Laura upstairs, and we both went to sleep happy and exhausted.

Thursday through Sunday

The next four days were quiet and uneventful. Laura spent most of her time sleeping. She did not eat much, except for an occasional teaspoon or two of ice cream, and I had been giving her ice chips to try and keep her hydrated. Although we had a portable commode, she insisted on going into the bathroom. I spent most of each day sitting next to the bed reading or watching TV. The hospice nurse came on Friday, and said there wasn't much change. Her blood pressure and pulse were still strong.

It was getting harder to get Laura to swallow pills, so I switched to the liquid morphine and antianxiety medication. The dosage for her pain patch had also been increased. When it was time to change her patches on Saturday,

. . . .

it was difficult to get the old patches off. Because she was becoming dehydrated, her skin had become dry, and trying to remove the patches was causing her a lot of discomfort.

I put in a call to the on-call nurse and explained the situation to her. I asked if leaving the old patches on would be okay. She was concerned there might be some trace medication in the old patches and recommended that I try to remove them. Not wanting to cause any unnecessary pain, I called a friend of Laura's who is a nurse and asked her opinion. She said that any trace medication would be minimal, and agreed that leaving the old patches on would probably be okay.

Laura had several visitors over the weekend, and one was unexpected. Her graduate-school advisor, Dr. Dana Cable, came over on Sunday afternoon. Laura had completed her graduate studies in December, and one of her goals was to attend graduation ceremonies to be held in May and receive her master's diploma. He knew Laura's condition was deteriorating, and he had a surprise for her. Realizing she was not going to make it to graduation, he had the college order her diploma and had it sent to him. He wanted to deliver it to her himself.

Laura recognized Dana when he walked into the room, and she smiled. He told her he had something for her and held the diploma for her to see. It took her a moment to focus on it, and when she realized what it was, she broke into a wide smile.

Monday

Early Monday morning I was awakened by the sound of banging. I thought it was someone knocking on the front door. I realized Laura was not in bed and ran downstairs. All the lights were out. Laura was in the kitchen standing near the refrigerator. She was banging a hard laminated placemat on the island. She had obviously been trying to get my attention. I looked at the clock; it was almost 4:30 a.m. I was amazed she had gotten out of bed by herself and made her way downstairs without falling. She had been so quiet she hadn't even awakened the dog.

I had become attuned to Laura's movement at night, and I usually woke up whenever she stirred. I had been up about an hour earlier, and she had been sleeping soundly. I remember thinking, she was going to sleep through the night, and I let myself fall into a deep sleep.

I could tell she was too weak to go up the stairs to the bedroom, so I guided her to the sofa in the family room and got her as comfortable as possible, covering her with the blanket she kept on her recliner. We cuddled on the sofa until eight o'clock in the morning, when she thought she had enough energy to make it up to the bedroom. I had to carry her up the last few stairs. Exhausted and scared, I realized I could not let something like this happen again. I decided I would contact an agency and have an aide stay for the overnight hours.

The rest of Monday quietly passed. Our friend, Julia, stayed most of the day, so I passed the day in the bedroom with Laura. The nurse came and was shocked when I told her about the previous night's adventure. In her words, "A guardian angel must have taken her down the stairs." Although Laura was very weak, her vital signs were still good. Sue told me she had noticed changes in Laura and thought it would be a few days at most.

The overnight home health aide arrived at 9 p.m. She would stay until 6 a.m. Tuesday and we planned to follow that routine each night. I set up a baby monitor in the den so the aide could hear any noise in the bedroom. We agreed that if Laura had to get up, the aide would come in and make sure things were okay. I felt sure there would be no repeat of the previous night.

Tuesday

I was dreading Tuesday. It was moving day for Willy. I had to be at his apartment in Washington, D.C. by 9 a.m. to meet the movers who were coming to move him from his apartment at the Westchester to Grand Oaks Assisted Living. I knew that even if things went perfectly, I would be gone for at least five to six hours. I wasn't worried about leaving Laura because she was in good hands. Robin, Kathy and Nancy, hospice friends, were going to take turns staying with her. More than anything else, I truly wanted to be at home at Laura's side in case something happened. In the previous two weeks, I hadn't been gone longer than an hour, and I just didn't want to be gone for a long period of time.

. . . .

Getting Willy into assisted living was a priority for Laura. We had been taking care of him since Laura's mother passed away in 1998. Although he lived on his own, his ability to manage basic daily tasks was limited. We managed his finances, paid his bills, and used an Internet service to have groceries delivered weekly. We had a maid service clean his apartment, and arranged for a home health aide to visit three times a week to do light housekeeping, laundry and cooking.

The idea of Willy moving to assisted living had been brought up with him and his doctor before Laura was diagnosed. Everyone except Willy thought it would be beneficial for him. When we knew Laura was dying, we spoke at length with Willy about the idea of moving, and he slowly warmed up to it. I think he agreed in part because he knew she was dying. Laura was concerned not only for Willy's future, but also for mine. She knew I would always be there for Willy, but having him in assisted living would take much of the burden from me.

Robin arrived at 7:30 a.m. Tuesday morning. I briefed her on the medication schedule and dosages, and I gave her a list of every possible phone number where she could reach me. I was on the road by 8 a.m.

Everything went as smoothly as possible. The movers showed up on time, and by 11 a.m. we had everything moved into his new residence. The brand-new furniture we bought a few weeks earlier was already in place. He and I spent an hour unpacking things and trying to get organized before we went to lunch in the dining room.

Over lunch, I told Willy that Laura wasn't doing well and she would probably die soon. I asked him if he wanted to come visit her, and he replied, "No. I'd rather remember her as she was." We agreed that he would call me every evening just to check in. He offered to help in any way possible, thanked me for taking such good care of her, and told me that he would be there for me.

I got back home around 2 p.m. Nancy was sitting in the bedroom while Laura slept. She told me everything had gone well, and Laura was comfortable and had slept most of the time. I was relieved and glad to be home.

I went up and sat with Laura. I told her everything had gone well, and Willy had told me he was sure he was going to like it there. I told her all the furniture fit, and Willy loved his new queen-sized bed. She didn't say much, but I knew she was relieved we had Willy settled in.

Dr. Meyer stopped in to check on Laura. He told me it would only be several more days. He told me that although he was going out of town on Wednesday, I was to call him if anything happened.

John came over and brought dinner. The first thing he did was to go up and see Laura. Over dinner, John told me that based on his experience with Vickie, his wife who had died, he thought the end was near.

Wednesday

Laura woke up around 4 a.m. on Wednesday. She was restless and trying to get comfortable. I gave Laura her medication, and she seemed to calm down, but never really went back to sleep. Two hours later she began to get restless again. I noticed her breathing was shallow, so I turned on the oxygen. This seemed to help a little, but she was not relaxed. I gave Laura another half-dose of medication, and she finally fell asleep. Around 7:30 a.m. the same thing began to happen. I called hospice and asked for the on-call nurse to call, and also for Sue, the regular nurse, to call.

The on-call nurse told me to give Laura another half dose of morphine, and if necessary to increase the frequency of doses. Sue called a little bit later, and I told her I was certain Laura was dying. She said she would make Laura her first visit of the day and would be here by 10 a.m.

I did my best to keep Laura comfortable, sitting by the bed, holding her hand. The additional medication was working, and she seemed to be comfortable. When Julia arrived, I quickly filled her in and went back to stay with Laura.

Sue arrived shortly before 10 o'clock followed by Helena, the home health aide, a few minutes later. Sue took Laura's vitals. Laura's blood pressure was low and respiration was shallow. Sue had a hard time getting a pulse. She told me Laura was dying, and it wouldn't be much longer.

I sat on the side of the bed holding her hand, telling her it was okay to go. I kissed her for the last time, told her I loved her and thanked her for a wonderful life. I promised I would take care of Gracie and Willy—and myself.

Laura took her last breath at 10:30 a.m.

. . . .

12

Unprepared

Although I knew that Laura was going to die, I wasn't prepared for it. There is no way you really can be. I was so numb. I couldn't even cry.

I stayed with Laura while the hospice nurse called Dr. Meyer to advise him that Laura had died. In Maryland, if a patient is under the care of a medical hospice, the hospice nurse can pronounce the patient deceased; there is no requirement to contact the police, paramedics or the coroner, as might be in other jurisdictions. I called the funeral home to come and get Laura, and because we had made prearrangements, all of the necessary paperwork was already on file.

I was with Julia and the hospice nurse waiting for the funeral home to come and get Laura. I called John and Nancy shortly after Laura died, and they both immediately came to the house. They both took charge of different things—John making some phone calls to friends, and the ever practical and maternal Nancy taking Julia out to get lunch for us.

I Sat There in a Fog

It was a surreal moment where things were going on around me, but I felt totally disconnected.

After the funeral home took Laura and the nurse left, it was just the four of us. We had lunch and talked about planning for the next several days. I had an appointment to go to the funeral home the next morning to finalize arrangements. John suggested I ask my friend, Brian, to go with me because he knew I would need someone with me for emotional support.

• •

Later that afternoon everyone left, and for the first time, Gracie and I were alone. I sat on the floor with Gracie in my lap and cried. It was starting to hit me. Later that evening, John and I went out for dinner. I went to bed when I got home, alone for the first time in 15 years. Through sheer exhaustion, I slept through the night.

Brian met me at the funeral home Thursday morning. It was a good thing he came along. Despite the prearrangements, I sat there as the funeral director went over things. Every time he asked me a question, I looked at Brian. I was having a tough time making the simplest decisions, such as what prayer cards did I want, and what verse did I want printed on the back of them. When we finally completed everything, there was one task left to do. I had to formally identify Laura's body for cremation.

The director led me to a viewing room and told me to take all the time I wanted. I had been dreading this moment and steeled myself to enter the room. Although Laura did not want a public viewing, they had her laid out in her casket in a small viewing room. I knelt by the casket and just stared at her. I couldn't believe that it was really her, and she was gone. The finality was beginning to hit me. I just knelt there and cried.

The week between when Laura died and her memorial service is a blur. The phone rang constantly, the daily mail was full of sympathy cards, and people were dropping by to offer their condolences. There were many details to be handled, and staying busy helped me get through those days.

The memorial service went smoothly. The turnout at the church was large. Laura had been afraid that no one would show up, and although I knew her fears were unfounded, I was amazed by the number of colleagues and students from Hood College, most of whom I had never met. I began to wonder if the room at the restaurant I had reserved for a reception after the service was going to be large enough.

The service was extremely emotional. The priest had asked me if I wanted to deliver a eulogy. Knowing that I would not be able to do it, I asked Kathy Ramsperger if she would speak. She and Laura had been friends since before I came along, and Kathy and Brian introduced us. Kathy delivered a wonderful

• • • • • • • • • • • • • • • • • • • •

tribute to Laura capturing the essence of her being and her passion for life. I was glad it wasn't me at the altar speaking. The mass ended with the priest reading the dedication of cousin Sara's doctoral dissertation:

> When I was a child you taught me to value family, pets, and people (especially boyfriends) who do the same. When I was an adult you taught me the history of our family and reminded me to live life to its fullest because it is so short. Thank you for being a wonderful role model, caring friend, keeper of family stories, a brilliant writer, and finding the strength to leave a legacy of help and hope for terminally ill cancer patients. I miss you.

The reception afterward was a welcome relief. It reminded me of the Italian wakes in New York. They were happy affairs, meant to celebrate the life of the deceased rather than death. It was comforting to spend time with family and friends who had come from as far as New York, Vermont and Seattle.

◆ ◆ ◆ ◆ ◆ ◆ ◆ ◆ ◆ ◆ ◆ ◆ ◆ ◆ ◆ ◆ ◆ ◆

13

On My Own

"I need to get back to normal, whatever that is, and I can't do that if you're here," I told Dad when he offered to stay longer. As much as I would have loved the comfort of having him in the house, I knew it would only delay the inevitable. I was going to have to live alone at some point. I had to figure out what my life was going to be and face that reality. I needed to go back to work and reestablish a routine for myself, so Dad went back to Florida the Saturday after the funeral.

I have been told it isn't until after the funeral is over and everyone goes back to his or her life that the reality really sets in. There is a lot of wisdom in that statement. I was now starting a new phase in my life. Being alone was going to be the norm. After the last several months of always having people around and being constantly busy, it was just me.

I have found similarities between what Laura went through, and to a lesser extent I went through, when she was first diagnosed. For the first two weeks after her death, I felt as if I were in a fog. I couldn't concentrate. I had no interest in anything and felt entirely lost and alone. Unless I was having dinner with friends, meals were unimportant. I had no desire to cook, and dinner became things like frozen pizza or take-out fast food. I had minimal interest in food, and eating was just another task.

During this period my emotions ran from anger to despair. I couldn't believe Laura had died and didn't want to accept it. I wasn't angry with her for dying, but I was angry at the fact she had died. The thought of being alone from now on was very unsettling.

I would ask myself "Who is going to take care of me?" My self-confidence was at an all time low, and I questioned every decision I made, even though they were only minor ones. I was forgetful. Many times, I would have to drive

· · · · · · · · · · · · · · · · · · · ·

back to the house and double check to make sure I did things like close the garage door or make sure I had put down fresh water for Gracie. I was physically and emotionally exhausted.

Establishing a new routine was my first goal. I had to think about things I never thought about before. I would be going back to work on Monday, so I had to make arrangements for Gracie. With Laura working from home, Gracie was used to having someone in the house for at least part of the day. She also needed medication and a meal at noon each day. My sleeping habits changed. I was waking up around 4 a.m., and that gave me time in the morning to walk the dog before I went to work. Julia was going to come three days a week and give Gracie her pills and meal, and walk her. The other two days, I would have to come home at lunchtime and take care of Gracie. Weekends wouldn't be a problem.

Going back to work was a welcome relief. It occupied a good part of my day, and there were a lot of people around. It took a few weeks for me to get back into the swing of things. My productivity was marginal at best, and it was hard to concentrate. Evenings and weekends were the hardest for me. Once I got home from work, time went into slow motion. I would pass the time by reading or watching television, but I really didn't have an interest in anything.

Weekends also became equally tough. I had a lot of time on my hands, but I had no inclination to do anything constructive with it. I had begun playing golf with John and his regular Sunday players. It was an excuse to get out of the house, but my heart wasn't in it—and it showed in the quality of my game.

I was getting a lot of support from friends and family, and I was reluctant to tell most of them how I was really doing. I would tell my closest friends "If I'm doing half as good as I want you to believe I am, then I'm doing okay." The last seven months had left me physically and emotional drained. I had lost 30 pounds—most of them in the last six weeks of Laura's illness.

Peoples' interaction with me since Laura's death has been very similar to their interaction with Laura during her illness. Professional friends of Laura that I didn't know before have kept in constant contact. I have received phone calls, emails and cards from them and invitations to have dinner with them. There is the core group of people that remains in constant contact.

• • • • • • • • • • • • • • • • • •

On the other hand, there are some longtime friends that I haven't heard from since she passed away. These are friends who were absent during Laura's illness, came to the memorial service and have once again disappeared.

One set of neighbors is a good example of how people's reactions and behavior can change in the face of adversity. Until the time that Laura was diagnosed, we had a reasonably close relationship with them. We would acknowledge birthdays and holidays with small gifts and cards. And we made arrangements to watch over each other's houses and collect the mail during vacations. We traded house keys in the event of an emergency.

During Laura's illness, they would ask how she was doing if we ran into each other, but they rarely called, and when they did, it was usually to ask if everything was okay because they saw cars parked in the driveway and wanted to know if something had happened.

Interacting with people is awkward sometimes. Some people don't know what to say, so they say nothing. It does not mean that they don't care; they just don't know what to say, so the conversation is very superficial. There have been situations where others have said, "I don't know what to say." Others have said things I never expected, such as "How can you sleep in the bed your wife died in?" or "Why are you still wearing your wedding ring?"

Friends had been telling me that I did a great job. I had problems accepting comments like this, not because I felt I didn't do a good job, but because in my mind I did what I had to do and what I would expect of anyone else in my shoes. I had taken our wedding vows very seriously, and things like "for better or for worse, in sickness and in health" weren't empty promises. I still don't believe I did anything extraordinary or heroic—I just took the best possible care of someone that I truly loved, and a part of me died with her. Looking back, I cannot think of anything I wish I had or hadn't done, nor anything I would have done differently. I get a lot of comfort from this, and it has made my days a little easier. I believe this is the reason why I am comfortable being in our house.

I have often wondered if seeing Willy settled was the last thing Laura wanted before she died. Looking back, when she had her early morning incident in the kitchen, she was looking at the "family schedule" calendar when I entered the room. Was she checking to see when the move was scheduled?

* *

As the days passed, I began to slowly put things in perspective. I realized that I had every reason to feel good about Laura's death. I had been able to give her the best final gift I possibly could—the good death that she had hoped for. Everything she wanted to happen did happen. Laura had died at home in her own bed with me there, and I don't believe she was in pain.

Things began to clarify further the night the updated *Nightline* program aired. A few days after Laura's death, Dan Green, the producer, called me to ask if I would consider doing a follow-up interview that they would incorporate into the original piece and run it again. My original thought was, "NO WAY." I really didn't think I had the strength to do it. I was also fairly sure I would not be able to do it with out breaking down. As I thought about it, I realized I was being given an opportunity to get Laura's message out again and agreed to do it.

Dan asked if there was anyone who could provide meaningful insight into Laura's death, and I immediately recommended John Driscoll and Nancy Ochsenreiter. They were both very involved in the last weeks of Laura's life and would offer two unique perspectives. John has been my friend seemingly forever and was the best man at our wedding. His wife, Vickie, had died several years ago after a seven-year battle with brain cancer. Nancy had the insight of being a close friend of Laura's as well as a hospice professional. We did the interviews on a Monday, and although Dan told me I did well, I didn't remember a word I said until I saw the program.

Watching the program was weird. I was seeing Laura and hearing her voice for the first time since she died. Even though she and I had watched the original broadcast several times before, watching it now was a different experience. Laura's words had taken on a new meaning. Her strength, courage and determination to get her message across were astounding. I began to realize that we had gone though a lifetime of emotions in a seven-month period. Although it was emotional to watch, when it was over I felt a sense of peace and calm that I hadn't felt in a long time. I had begun to understand what people meant when they said I did a good job.

There is no formula for grieving. It is a process that evolves over time. Because I can talk about Laura without crying doesn't mean I'm not grieving. I miss her all the time. I often talk to her just to tell her about something that happened. Or, I tell her how good her gardens looked this spring. Many things are constant reminders of her.

I am finding the key to moving forward is keeping busy. The best advice I was given came from my father. Shortly before he left, he said, "Don't do what I'm doing. Do something with your life." My parents had been married for 52 years when my mother died. They had a very strong marriage that weathered many adversities, including the accident that disabled Dad in 1959, Mom's breast cancer in the 1960s, and the death of a daughter-in-law, Mary Ellen, whom they considered a daughter. For the last 10 years of her life, Mom had Alzheimer's disease. Dad had cared for her at home until it became physically impossible for him to continue. She spent the last two years of her life in a nursing home where he would visit her every day.

When Mom died, Dad was devastated. Suddenly he had no purpose in life. Despite the urgings of my brother, John, and me, along with other family members, he was reluctant to move on with his life. He was content to stay home and fell into a routine of mundane activities to fill his days. Unless it was a trip to visit Laura and me, or John and Amy, he rebuffed our suggestions to travel. It seemed ironic that the advice to "do something with my life" came from him.

I believe that coming to Maryland to help take care of Laura helped him to deal with his pain of losing Mom. He was helping us, and by doing that he was helping himself. It gave him a purpose in life that had been missing. His outlook has changed, and he recently decided to take a trip to Hawaii with his brother.

Grieving does not mean that you are not allowed to have fun. Laura and I had many talks about my being alone after she died. She had told me that she expected me to continue with life. She had talked to our friends about making sure I would be okay. She did not want me to sit around and be depressed and do nothing. She expected me to live, not merely exist; however, I did feel guilty at times for attending a party or going out with friends.

Gradually, the idea of keeping busy has evolved from merely passing time to enjoying that time or being productive. When I first started playing golf after Laura died, it was merely a means to kill time and get out of the house. Now, I look forward to the Sunday golf games and enjoy being with my friends.

* * * * * * * * * * * * * * * *

As a result of this, my golf game has improved. At John's urging, I am also playing in a Tuesday night golf league. I have also begun to make travel plans for later in the year, and I made a quick trip out west to attend my goddaughter's college graduation and visit my nephew.

One of the key factors to my recovering from Laura's death has been the support of family and friends. There is a core group of people that has made it their personal mission to make sure I'm dealing with things. It has given me the opportunity to talk about Laura. Sometimes I vent my frustration and anger to the point where the conversations have been like therapy. I cannot fully express my gratitude to them. I am truly blessed to be surrounded by such supportive and giving friends. External resources are also available. The hospice that helped with Laura's care offers bereavement and grief counseling, and local organizations like Hospice Caring also offer grief counseling. I have also spoken with the priest who performed the memorial services.

Getting back to a normal life has also meant taking care of myself. I have begun to catch up on things that I put on hold while I was taking care of Laura. I now have the time to schedule overdue dentist and doctor appointments. These are all signs that I am moving forward.

Gracie

Gracie was also affected by Laura's death. She had been a wonderful companion for Laura during her illness. In the final weeks when Laura spent most of her time in bed, Gracie often spent hours at a time lying on the floor next to the bed.

After everyone left the house the day Laura died, Gracie went looking for "Mom." She didn't know Laura wasn't coming back, and she spent the better part of the next several weeks lying by the front door waiting for her. She would wander through the house as if she were looking for Laura. Although Gracie had normally slept on the floor in our bedroom, for almost two weeks after Laura died, she slept by the front door.

In many ways, Gracie's behavior mirrored my own. She was nervous, and she showed minimal interest in anything, including eating and playing. She would reluctantly go for a walk but did not want to go too far from the house. As the weeks passed, she began to act more like her old self.

* * * * * * * * * * * * * * * * * * * *

14

Looking Back

Wednesday, May 5, 2004: Today is my 50th birthday. I haven't felt this alone since the day Laura died. It's hard to believe that it's been only 70 days since she passed away. In some ways it seems like yesterday, but in other ways it seems like it has been years.

It's only 7 a.m., and I've already cried three times. Too many memories are rushing back. I missed Laura singing "Happy Birthday" as only she could, and the birthday cards from Laura and Gracie sitting on the kitchen table when I came downstairs to have my morning coffee.

The one goal that Laura had that she didn't make was to be here today. She wanted to make my 50th birthday "special" as a payback for the 50th birthday party I had thrown for her. I chartered *Woodwind*, a 72-foot schooner, for a birthday cruise and lunch. We loaded 25 friends and relatives on a chartered bus for the trip to Annapolis and spent four hours sailing on the Chesapeake Bay. We ended the day with a party back at the house.

In contrast, I want this day to go by as quickly as possible, and with as little attention as possible. I have declined invitations from Brian and Kathy, Robin, Nancy and Glenn because I'm not in a celebratory mood. I'm also afraid it would be too painful for me to be with them because of their close relationship with Laura and me. Instead, I am having dinner with my boss, Linda, and some friends from work. They are wonderful people to be around, and they have been very supportive. Most of them didn't know Laura, so I'm hoping that dinner will be less emotional.

When I got home from work there was a gift on the island in the kitchen. I knew it was from Julia. There were two cards—one from her and another from Gracie. They really made me feel good.

. . . .

Dinner was exactly as I hoped it would be. The conversation was light and the topics were casual. I was able to enjoy dinner, and when I got home I was in pretty good spirits. I was confident I would make it through the rest of the evening okay. I had survived my birthday.

Laura's Graduation

Saturday, May 22, 2004, was Laura's graduation date. Getting her "Master of Arts—Thanatology" degree, the study of death and dying, from Hood College, was one of her proudest accomplishments. I had decided to attend the commencement exercises, and when her advisor, Dr. Dana Cable, asked me if I wanted to participate by ceremoniously accepting her diploma, I felt it would be a fitting tribute to her.

I asked Dad to come up and spend a few days and attend the graduation with me. I also decided to throw a party that evening to celebrate Laura's memory and to a lesser extent acknowledge my birthday.

Dad and I arrived at the graduation and were given seats in the second row. I was right on the aisle where the graduates would be lining up next to me. I would be told when to take my place in line. I was instructed to take my cues from the person in front of me. As I was waiting for the ceremony to start, I gave myself a pep talk. I knew it was going to be an emotional moment, and I was trying to convince myself that I could do this without breaking down. It wasn't supposed to be like this. I had always envisioned Laura walking up to receive her degree, with a very proud me sitting in the audience.

The commencement exercise started, and I watched carefully. It would be a short walk to the stage, up the stairs and a few more steps to where the Hood College President, Ronald J. Volpe, was handing out the diplomas. A quick handshake and then another quick shake of the hand from Dr. Regina Lightfoot, graduate school dean, off the stage and back to my seat. It would take less than two minutes. I could handle this.

Laura's name was announced, and I headed up the stairs and walked to the president. I accepted her diploma, and I began to step away. He told me to wait and turn toward the audience. They paused the commencement, and the dean of graduate students read a tribute to Laura. I was so overcome with emotion

· · · · · · · · · · · · · · · · · ·

that I stood there unable to hear the words being spoken. As I walked off the stage, I realized that the entire crowd of graduates, faculty, parents and guests was standing and applauding.

After the ceremony, Dad and I attended the graduate student reception. We sat with several of Laura's professors and fellow students. At the end of the reception, they wanted to have a quick ceremony in Laura's memory. We stood in a circle and Norval Kennedy, a classmate of Laura's and a writer and editor, explained that they would pass a graduation tassel and each one would say something about Laura. I began crying as Norval began speaking, and I didn't stop until the tassel was passed to me. I was barely able to thank them for their kind remembrances.

Dad and I were silent on the ride home. I replayed the event in my mind and thought back to Dr. Volpe's address to the graduates. He had spoken about the graduates reaching a turn in their life's path that would take them to new and unknown experiences. In many ways his speech applied to me. When Laura died I was on the path alone for the first time in 15 years and had come to a turn. I don't know what lies ahead, but like the students, I am optimistic.

The party that evening proved to be the perfect counterbalance to the graduation ceremony. This day was full of emotion, and having friends and family around brightened my mood. This was the first time since Laura's funeral that we had all gotten together. Everyone who was there had played an important role in our lives, and it proved to be a fitting and happy tribute to Laura.

• •

15

One Day at a Time

The tension is slowly building again. There are several milestone days ahead, and I am approaching them with a sense of dread. I have been told the first special occasion or holiday after a loved one dies is the hardest to deal with, and I should expect days like this to be especially difficult. I have also been told that the anticipatory grief in the days leading up to that special day can be worse than the day itself.

I had my first meltdown, after feeling comparatively stable for a few weeks, on the Fourth of July. I had played golf that morning and was just sitting at home relaxing when all of a sudden I was overwhelmed. Laura's birthday was coming up on the seventh, and the day after that was the first anniversary of the day she was diagnosed. To top things off, July 9th will be the 16th anniversary of the day we met.

I think of what would have occurred had things been different, and the memories come rushing back. We would be going to the Homestead to celebrate Laura's birthday. I can imagine us sitting in the President's Lounge having a predinner cocktail and sitting on the balcony of our room watching the sunset over the golf course. I remember the fun we had when I would play golf and Laura would drive the cart, and the leisurely lunch we would have on the Casino porch afterwards. Although these thoughts are painful, they are also comforting.

Laura's Birthday

Today is Laura's birthday. I have been thinking of her constantly. It is very hard to believe that she is gone. I can see a subtle distinction between the way I feel today as opposed to the way I felt on my birthday in May. The sense of loneliness and loss are as deep as they were then, but the feelings of total despair have diminished.

• •

Today is also significant for another reason. It is the first anniversary of the last "normal" day of our lives. Although Laura was in considerable pain, we were blissfully unaware of the underlying cause, and we honestly believed that whatever the problem, it was treatable. We had no idea that in less than 24 hours our world would explode with the delivery of a death sentence for Laura and our lives would be forever changed. It's hard to believe it has been a year.

I continue to make positive strides in my grief. My outlook on things is becoming more positive. I am finding enjoyment in things, and I am able to relax. I am comfortable at home, and have settled into a relatively normal routine. I am taking life one day at a time.

The one thing that has helped me the most in the last few months has been completing this book. The one question that people kept asking me was, "What about the book?" Laura began writing this book to help others. It was her goal to complete it, but that wasn't meant to be. I had promised her I would be sure that it was finished. I had been reluctant to look at it for several reasons, the primary one being that I wasn't emotionally prepared to spend a lot of time in her office. The second reason was the more frightening one—I am not a writer. I had no idea how to even begin to finish her work.

The inspiration came to me after a conversation with one of our friends, Denise, the hospice professional in Frederick, Maryland. She told me her sister-in-law had recently been diagnosed with brain cancer. Denise was having an extremely difficult time coping with this. "I am dealing with her illness on a professional level because I can't deal with it on an emotional level," she told me. Having been through Laura's illness, I could relate to what she was saying.

The next day, I awoke with a vision for the book mapped out. I realized this book needed to be the book I wished I had been able to find when Laura was first diagnosed, a kind of "been there, done that" book that documented things from the perspective of the patient *and* the caregiver. Finishing this book has been cathartic for me. It has been painful at times to revisit the bad moments, but it also made me remember the good things that sometimes get overlooked.

There are a lot of things I haven't done yet. There is no need to hurry. I have been advised not to make any major decisions for a while. This makes a lot of sense. I don't want to make any decisions that might seem appropriate at the time, but I might regret later. This includes going through Laura's things. At some point in the future I will go through her office and her clothing.

* * * * * * * * * * * * * * * * * *

A part of my life is gone and will never be replaced. Laura had always said we were the perfect team because our outlook on things struck a balance. She tended to look at the glass as being half empty, and I looked at it as being half full. This outlook has helped me in my grief. I am very grateful for what we did have. Fifteen years is not a long time, but I believe in that period of time we had achieved something that some people never do. We were soul mates, and she will be a part of me forever. I am not the most religious person in the world, but I do believe in God, and I believe that the soul is eternal. I am certain that Laura and I will eventually be reunited. It is a very comforting thought.

I met a man at a hospice event recently who lost his wife two years ago. He offered me encouragement and support. He recently assured me that although I might not be able to see it now, there really is a light at the end of the tunnel. Every once in a while, I can see it flickering.

* * * * * * * * * * * * * * * * * *

References

Chapter 2

1. American Cancer Society (2003). *Pancreatic Cancer.* Austin, TX, p. 3.

Chapter 4

1. Clark, J. (2003). Patient Centred Death. *British Medical Journal*, 327: p. 174-175. July 26th Edition.
2. Institute of Medicine (2003). *Approaching Death: Improving Care At The End of Life.* Washington, DC: National Academy Press. p. 24.
3. Steinhauser, K.E., Christakis, N.A., Clipp, E.C., McNeilly M, McIntyre, L. Tulsky, J.A. (2000). Factors considered important at the end of life by patients, family, physicians, and other care providers. *Journal of the American Medical Association*, 284: p. 2476-2782.
4. Teno, J.M., Clarridge, B.R., Casey, V., Welch, L.C., Wetle T., Shield, R., Mor, V. (2004). Family Perspectives on End-of-Life Care at the Last Place of Care. *Journal of the American Medical Association*, 291: pp. 88-93.
5. Corr, C.A., Nabe, C.M., Corr, D.M. (2000). *Death and Dying. Life and Living.* Belmont, CA: Wadsworth/Thomson Learning, p. 148.

Chapter 5

1. Saunders, Y., Ross, J.R., Riley, J. (2003). Planning for a good death: responding to unexpected events. *British Medical Journal*, 327:204-206.
2. American Cancer Society (2003). *Pancreatic Cancer*, Austin, TX, p. 3.
3. American Cancer Society (2003). *Cancer Facts & Figures.* Austin, TX, p. 4.
4. American Cancer Society (2003). *Cancer Facts & Figures.* Austin, TX, p. 2
5. Institute of Medicine (1997). *Approaching Death. Improving Care At The End of Life.* Washington, DC: National Academy Press, p. 126.

Chapter 6

1. Nuland, S.B. (1994). *How We Die: Reflections on Life's Final Chapter.* New York, NY: Alfred K. Knopf, p. 221.
2. Ibid, p. 221.
3. Gottlieb, S. (2001). Chemotherapy may be overused at the end of life. *British Medical Journal*, 322:1267.

◆ ◆ ◆ ◆ ◆ ◆ ◆ ◆ ◆ ◆ ◆ ◆ ◆ ◆ ◆ ◆ ◆

4. Rosenbaum, E.H., Rosenbaum, I. (2001). *Supportive Cancer Care: The Complete Guide for Patients and Their Families.* Naperville, IL; Sourcebooks, Inc., p. 231.

Chapter 7
1. House, A., Stark, D. (2002) Anxiety in Medical Patients. *British Medical Journal*, 325: 207-209.
2. Paice, J.A. (2002). Managing Psychological Conditions in Palliative Care, *American Journal of Nursing*, Vol. 102, No. 11, pp. 38–39.
3. Ibid, p. 38
4. Lynn, J. & Harrold, J. (1999). *Handbook for Mortals. Guidance for People Facing Serious Illness.* New York: Oxford University Press, p. 91.
5. Corr, C.A., Nabe, C.M., Corr, D.M. (2000). *Death and Dying. Life and Living.* Belmont, CA: Wadsworth/ Thomson Learning, p. 165.
6. Paice, J.A. (2002). Managing Psychological Conditions in Palliative Care, *American Journal of Nursing*, Vol. 102, No. 11, pp. 39.
7. National Cancer Institute (2004). Depression PDQ (Assessment and Diagnosis). Bethesda, MD; National Institutes of Health, p. 4.
8. Byock, I. (1997). *Dying Well: Peace and Possibilities at the End of Life.* New York: Riverhead Books, p. 101.
9. National Cancer Institute (2004). Depression PDQ (Overview). Bethesda, MD; National Institutes of Health, p. 2.
10. Lloyd-William. M., Dennis, M., Taylor, F. Baker, I. (2003). Is asking patients in palliative care, "Are you depressed?" appropriate? Prospective study. *British Medical Journal*, 327: p. 372-376.
11. Christakis, N.A., Lamont, E.B. (2000). Extent and determinants of error in doctors' prognoses in terminally ill patients: prospective cohort study. *British Medical Journal*, 320: p. 469-471.
12. The, A., Hak, T., Koeter, G., van der Wal, G. (2000). Collusion in doctor-patient communication about imminent death: an ethnographic study. *British Medical Journal*, 321: p. 1376-1381.
13. Lynn, J., Harrold, J. (1999). *Handbook for Mortals: Guidance for People Facing Serious Illness.* New York: Oxford University Press, p. 94.
14. Weissman, D. (2000). Determining Prognosis in Advanced Cancer. End of Life/Palliative Education Resource Center, Fast Fact and Concept #013. Accessed at www.eperc.mcw.edu.
15. Institute of Medicine (1997). A*pproaching Death: Improving Care At The End of Life.* Washington, DC: National Academy Press, p. 23.

* * * * * * * * * * * * * * * * * * *

Resources

Administration on Aging. Fact sheet titled "Respite: What Caregivers Need Most" www.aoa.gov/factsheets/Respite.html; 202-619-0724

AllExperts. An online volunteer site with health professionals who answer questions about diseases, treatments, tests, finding care, death and dying. www.allexperts.com

Alzheimer's Association. Provides information, referrals, and support for patients and caregivers. www.alz.org; 800-272-3900

American Association of Homes and Services for the Aging (AAHSA). Information on over 5,600 nonprofit elder-care facilities. www.aahsa.org; 202-782-2242

American Association of Retired Persons. AARP has brochures dealing with many age-related issues like eldercare, end-of-life, and grief recovery. www.aarp.org; 800-424-3410.

American Cancer Society. For referrals, educational materials, and questions. www.cancer.org; 800-227-2345

American Diabetes Association. For referrals, educational materials, and questions. www.diabetes.org; 800-342-2383

American Heart Association. For referrals, educational materials, and questions. www.americanheart.org; 800-242-8721

Hospice Foundation of America. Offers a national database of hospice providers. www.hospicefoundation.org; 800-854-3402

Law and Aging Resource Guide. State-by-state directory of legal resources and services for seniors published by the American Bar Association. www.abanet.org; 202-662-8690

Medicare Rights Center. Information on Medicare coverage. www.medicarerights.org; 212-869-3850

National Hospice & Palliative Care Organization (NHPCO). Provides over 22,000 resources for people seeking hospice or home care. Offers brochures. www.nhpco.org; 800-646-6460

National Institutes of Health (NIH). National clearinghouse for medical research with extensive information search capabilities. www.nih.gov/nia; 800-438-4380

• •

Medications

_____

_____

_____

_____

_____

_____

_____

_____

_____

_____

_____

_____

_____

_____

_____

_____

_____

_____

_____

_____

_____

* * * * * * * * * * * * * * * * * * *

Contacts

_____
_____
_____
_____
_____
_____
_____
_____
_____
_____
_____
_____
_____
_____
_____
_____
_____
_____
_____
_____
_____
_____

* * * * * * * * * * * * * * * * * * *

Notes

_____

_____

_____

_____

_____

_____

_____

_____

_____

_____

_____

_____

_____

_____

_____

_____

_____

_____

_____

_____

_____

_____

_____

_____

_____

* * * * * * * * * * * * * * * * * * * *

Notes

_____

_____

_____

_____

_____

_____

_____

_____

_____

_____

_____

_____

_____

_____

_____

_____

_____

_____

_____

_____

_____

_____

_____

_____

_____

_____

◆ ◆